If Your Child Has Diabetes

If Your Child Has Diabetes

An Answer Book for Parents

JOANNE ELLIOTT

A PERIGEE BOOK

Perigee Books
are published by
The Putnam Publishing Group
200 Madison Avenue
New York, NY 10016

The information contained in this book is the result of a careful review of the medical literature. However, new information is constantly becoming available and individual responses to specific treatments, methods, and medications vary widely from person to person. The reader should consult with his or her physician before acting on any of the information contained herein. The author and publisher specifically disclaim responsibility for any adverse effect or unforeseen consequences resulting from the implementation of any information mentioned in this book.

Library of Congress Cataloging-in-Publication Data

Elliott, Joanne, date.
If your child has diabetes : an answer book for parents / by
Joanne Elliott.
p. cm.
Includes bibliographical references.
1. Diabetes in children—Popular works. 2. Diabetes in children—
Patients—Care. I. Title.
RJ420.D5E45 1990 89–29041 CIP
618.92′462—dc20
ISBN 0-399-51610-7

Printed in the United States of America
1 2 3 4 5 6 7 8 9 10

This book has been printed on acid-free paper.

Acknowledgments

I am grateful to Drs. Margery Meyers and Timothy Lyons and to Jenny Campbell, who brought me up to date with the American diabetic scene; also to Dr. Randall Hayes of the Belfast City Hospital, who is never too busy to help. I am indebted to Peter and Joan, who presented me with a wonderful word processor, to Susan, who cooked and cleaned while I scribbled, and to Eric, who put up with it all.

This book is dedicated to my family with love.

Did you know that . . .

girls with diabetes often menstruate later than their nondiabetic sisters?

people with diabetes should eat a low-fat diet?

children who cannot eat because of illness need more insulin, not less?

"freezing" the injection site with an ice cube can make shots less painful?

injecting dolls and stuffed toys helps a child to come to terms with diabetes?

Contents

Introduction *11*

Preface to the American Edition *13*

1 About Diabetes *17*

2 Insulin, Injections, and Reactions *29*

3 Control *54*

4 Food Plan *84*

5 School, Camp, and Exercise *122*

6 Emotional Problems *133*

7 Diabetes in the Very Young *139*

8 The Teen Years *147*

9 Traveling *164*

10 Medical Costs, Insurance, Research, and Development *170*

11 Special Treats *177*

Appendices *181*

1 Injection Sites *181*

2 Hypoglycemia (Low Blood Glucose) *182*

3 Hyperglycemia (High Blood Glucose) *183*

4 Diabetic Ketoacidosis (Very High Blood Glucose With Ketones) *184*

5 Some Books About Diabetes *185*

6 Useful Addresses *187*

Index *188*

Introduction

Some years ago, I was asked to speak to a group of parents whose children had developed diabetes. The topic I was given was "How Parents Can Help." Not knowing how to begin, I asked my daughter with diabetes, then about ten years old. Her answer was short and simple. "Parents can help," she declared, "by knowing everything."

No one can know everything about diabetes. There is so much that is yet to be discovered. We, as parents, though, can certainly make a start, for we start with the knowledge that the more we learn about this disease, the better we can control it.

I am a parent like you. The training I have had in diabetes has been on-the-job training, learning to cope with my child's daily life. You are learning now in the same way that I did, slowly and painfully. Many aspects of diabetes are frightening. No one wants to think about the complications that could arise in later life. Refusing to think about them, however, will not make them go away. On the contrary, learning to control this disease more effectively will reduce the possibility that your child will develop complications. Learning does more than promote better diabetic control. It also promotes better mental health. When a child is first diagnosed, it is a bitter blow. "Why me?" asks the child.

"Why my child?" ask the parents. Fear, guilt, and despair hold them fast.

The child is frightened to be different. The parents fear that they cannot cope with the demands that this condition will require. They feel depressed and helpless in the face of this unseen menace, this "fickle finger of fate" that has reached out from nowhere to threaten their family. But by mastering this fear and pain, by learning to control the disease instead of being controlled by it, parents learn to fight back. *It is a fight that can be won.*

The fact that you, the parent, are sitting here reading this book instead of collapsing into bed with nerves or emptying a bottle of spirits in the nearest cocktail lounge means that you have taken the first step. You have decided that you are not helpless. You and your child will learn. You will fight back and your life will be normal again. It is my aim to give you the necessary weapons so that you will win.

As a volunteer for the British Diabetic Association and in my work as a diabetic educator, I have spoken to hundreds of parents. We have discussed our mutual problems by the hour. As parents together, we talked about the things that we were too diffident to mention to the doctor or the nurse. We talked about the moodiness of the child with diabetes, about his fear of being "different." We talked about our dread of nighttime insulin reactions, about school and exam pressures, about difficult grandparents and well-meaning but thoughtless friends. Learning to cope with these problems is as important to your child's health as learning good injection techniques and counting exchanges.

In this book, I try to cover all aspects of diabetic care, physical and emotional, to supply as many answers as I can to the endless stream of questions that you, the parent, need to ask.

Preface to the American Edition

When the idea of producing an American edition was first suggested by my publishers, I agreed with alacrity. It would just be a matter of a few spelling changes, I thought, deleting references to the British Diabetic Association and the National Health Service, and Americanizing the food plan. It was only when I actually began working on the manuscript that the differences hit me. As they are fond of saying on the European side of the Atlantic, Britain and America are two countries divided by a common language.

The first problem I had to tackle was the medical one: who diagnoses the diabetes and how is it looked after from there? There is no room for debate or even choice in the UK. Anyone who goes to his doctor with insulin-dependent diabetes is immediately referred to the nearest hospital for admission, often the same day. If that hospital is a large teaching facility, he is lucky. There is a diabetic clinic staffed with specialists, nurses, dieticians, and a lab. The patient is stabilized in about a week and discharged with an appointment to return to the clinic every three months. He is also given a supply of insulin, syringes, urine- and blood-testing equipment, and a letter is sent to his family doctor with a request to give him prescriptions for refills whenever necessary.

The prescriptions can be filled free of charge at any pharmacy. If he should require a pen injector or even a pump in the future, this is usually given to him by the hospital clinic, the pump on indefinite loan, the pen a gift from the manufacturers. Diabetes education is supplied by the physicians and the diabetes nurse specialists. Occasionally, one comes across a diabetes educator. At necessary intervals, blood is sent to the lab, ophthalmic appointments are scheduled, and the diet sheet is updated. The patient is urged to join the British Diabetic Association (a medical-lay organization) and to attend a holiday camp or teaching weekend. This is the usual procedure for the patient who lives in or near a large urban center.

Those in the boondocks are less well looked after. Small cottage hospitals rarely have endocrinologists on the staff, and patients who express a desire to see one are usually discouraged. Asking for a second opinion is often construed as criticism. Unless you are a brash American like me, you generally put up with whatever the local medical scene has to offer, supplementing by joining the BDA and reading their magazine. Money never enters the picture. All medical care is dispensed free at the point of use. Everyone who works pays toward the National Health Service in the same way that Americans pay toward Social Security. Theoretically, everyone has a completely free choice of physicians; but on a practical basis, the choice is dictated by geography. The general practitioner will accept a new patient only in the area within which he makes home visits, and each GP has certain specialists to whom he likes to refer his patients. The quality of care available, then, is mostly a matter of luck, the poor and less educated getting the short end of the stick because they are less inclined to question anything and less able to take time off from work to travel to where the service is better.

In the UK and Ireland—probably in Europe as a whole—class structures are more rigid than in the United States. The doctor has enormous prestige. His word is law, especially in rural areas, and the patient is inclined to accept meekly whatever he is told. Lawsuits are so rare that they make the headlines.

Complications tend to be downplayed. Until a few years ago, material intended to be read by lay people, especially books and magazines for children with diabetes and their parents, hardly discussed the complications of diabetes at all. Today, the outlook is slightly more realistic, but on the whole, there is still a more casual attitude toward diabetes management. The American obsession with health is regarded here with some amusement. Still, for all that, fitness has begun to assume a larger place in people's consciousness. Fewer adults smoke; less meat, full-cream milk, and butter is consumed, and more people participate in regular exercise than was true twenty years ago. Few British or Irish people know anything about nutrition, a subject of little general interest until recently. The posters showing the "basic seven" foodstuffs that decorated the wall of every classroom I was in from kindergarten to the eighth grade is an American phenomenon. In my counseling work in a diabetic clinic, I had to start from scratch explaining to almost every patient or parent, even college graduates, what constitutes carbohydrate food. Food packages carry skimpy nutritional breakdowns, and putting together a suitable diet is sometimes difficult.

Emotional problems connected with diabetes are generally glossed over unless they are severe. A few centers have resident child psychologists, but this is the exception rather than the rule. Hospital staff expect that children of eight will be able to inject themselves after a few days and take a firm line in the matter. A stiff upper lip is encouraged, and, although advice is generally dispensed freely, patients and parents are expected to be uncomplaining. The word *adjustment* is not in common use.

It is interesting that the needle-free injectors advertised in every issue of American diabetes magazines are never seen in British ones. Whether this is purely a matter of economics or whether cultural attitudes have a part to play is a matter for speculation.

Life is less complicated for the British or Irish person with diabetes because he has fewer choices to make and because the cost of his treatment is spread among the working population. Should a very expensive new treatment become available, however, he may not be aware of it. Still, even those at the bottom of the economic scale receive adequate and often excellent treatment. Physicians in the forefront of diabetes research and care are a small and dedicated coterie.

Diet is generally simpler and less varied, as people here are less interested in food. The enormous range of sugarless, fat-free, and low-sodium manufactured foods that fill the shelves of every American supermarket would be a revelation and a delight.

Americans are conditioned to look after their health themselves. They tend to be more active, assertive, and knowledgeable in this regard. Perhaps having to buy medical care makes it an expensive commodity that is chosen carefully rather than one that is accepted with few questions.

No matter on which side of the Atlantic one lives, however, there is no doubt that contemporary diabetes care in the developed world has put the emphasis on the person himself. No longer is it the physician who prescribes and the patient who obeys. A partnership has developed within the established relationship. With the aid of the new technology, the patient himself collects the data that forms the basis of his medical advice. Not only does he collect the information, but, with the aid of the medical team, he interprets and acts upon it. He has virtually become his own physician. It is freely acknowledged that since it is the person with diabetes who must live with the disease, it is he who must learn enough to control it. Hence the importance of diabetes education, which goes hand in hand with sound medical advice. While the information in this book is intended to help you and your child understand diabetes and its treatment, it is not a substitute for the advice of your own doctor. An educated person with diabetes still needs to be under the regular treatment of a medical doctor, skilled in the treatment of diabetes.

1

About Diabetes

Q: *What exactly is diabetes?*
A: Diabetes, or diabetes mellitus (sugar diabetes), is a disorder of the means by which the body changes the food we eat into energy. This is a basic function of life. A person develops diabetes when this function is impaired, when there is insufficient insulin, or when the cells cannot use insulin properly.

Q: *Why is insulin important?*
A: If too little of the hormone insulin is produced by the pancreas, a gland that lies behind the stomach, too much glucose (a simple sugar) gathers in the blood. Without insulin to enable the cells to absorb it, the glucose from the food we eat has nowhere to go and accumulates in the bloodstream. When the level of glucose in the blood gets too high, it spills over into the urine, taking along large amounts of water and salts drawn from the cells. The early symptom of diabetes is frequent passing of urine, which, in turn, causes great thirst.

Q: *Is glucose the only substance affected?*
A: Other substances are controlled by insulin as well. These are fatty acids and amino acids. Glucose gives us quick energy; fatty

acids are stored for energy in the future and amino acids are the components of protein. Insulin directs these three substances through the body. Without sufficient insulin, the body cannot store reserves of glucose, protein, and fat, so rapid degeneration follows. Without insulin treatment, weight loss, dehydration, coma, and eventually death will result.

Q: *Why does the pancreas stop making insulin?*

A: The precise cause is unknown, but the latest scientific research indicates that diabetes is an autoimmune disease. The pancreas stops making insulin because the body destroys its own insulin-producing cells.

The insulin-producing cells, the beta cells, are found in the islets of Langerhans, which are clusters of cells scattered throughout the pancreas. (The islets of Langerhans also contain alpha cells, which make glucagon.) In certain people, the beta cells are attacked and destroyed by substances called islet-cell antibodies. The people whose beta cells are destroyed develop diabetes.

The tendency to produce islet-cell antibodies, often referred to as ICA, may be inherited. Not everyone, though, who has inherited a tendency to manufacture islet-cell antibodies will do so. Another factor may come into play that triggers off ICA production in a person with an inherited tendency to diabetes.

Q: *What is this other factor?*

A: There are indications that it might be a virus, probably a common one. This virus contains a substance identical to a substance in the beta cells of the islets of Langerhans. The body's immune system, programmed to destroy that particular substance in the virus, destroys it in the beta cells as well.

Q: *Could I have known that my child would react in this way to such a virus?*

A: No. At present, there is no way that you could have known this. The virus is most likely a common one that other members of the household may have suffered at the same time.

Q: *If I had brought my child to the doctor earlier, could the diabetes have been prevented?*
A: No. The earlier the condition is diagnosed, the less marked will be the symptoms, but the disease would still exist even if it were diagnosed on the first day.

Q: *Is there anything that I could have done to keep my child from developing diabetes?*
A: No. Nothing. The ability of the pancreas to produce insulin is probably diminished for many years in the susceptible person before he or she actually develops diabetes. The process of destruction of the islet cells by antibodies may begin at birth, possibly even before birth. Given the appropriate trigger, that process will be accelerated until insulin production becomes so feeble that diabetes will result.

Q: *Did I do anything to contribute to it? If I had fed him differently, perhaps prevented him from eating so much candy or drinking soda, would I have been able to prevent it?*
A: Nothing you did or failed to do has had the slightest effect on the fact that your child developed diabetes. Blaming yourself is very natural but completely unjustified.

Q: *If I had been more careful, could I have kept him from developing the particular virus that started it off?*
A: No one knows exactly what the virus is. In fact, the virus theory is still only a theory. Genetic factors play a part as well, and there are many other factors that are not understood. A recent study shows that a Finnish child is seventeen times more likely to develop diabetes than a Japanese child and three times more likely than a California child.

Q: *Will my child outgrow his diabetes?*
A: I wish I could tell you that he would, but unfortunately, it isn't true. He will always have diabetes. I was plagued, in the first few years after my child developed the disease, by well-meaning

friends who assured me that she would outgrow it. It is not possible. Not only will your child always have diabetes, but if he has Type 1 diabetes, he will always need insulin. There are no wonder cures in diabetes, and you should beware of anyone who tells you that there are. Be skeptical of miracles and examine any nonmedical approaches as probably quackery.

Q: *At what age can children develop diabetes?*
A: At any age. Most children who develop diabetes do so during the school years, but it can develop much earlier. Although rare, it can happen in infancy, even soon after birth.

Q: *Can diabetes be cured?*
A: At the moment, there is no cure for diabetes. There has been so much research in this area, however, that it is possible that a cure will be found in the not-too-distant future.

Q: *Now that one of my children has developed diabetes, will the others become diabetic as well?*
A: Statistically, less than 5 percent of the brothers and sisters of a person with Type 1 diabetes develop the disease (assuming that the parents do not have diabetes). The number of families with more than one member with diabetes is small.

Q: *Can diabetes be prevented?*
A: Recently, work has been done to identify children at risk, with a view toward prevention. This work, which involves tissue typing and detailed studies of the genetic makeup of the cells, is still in its early stages. In the future, however, it might be possible to prevent the development of diabetes in a susceptible person by reprogramming a part of the immune system. This would mean targeting other antibodies to remove the ones that might destroy the beta cells. As you can imagine, this is enormously complicated, but many medical researchers are confident that it can be done. So much more is now understood about diabetes that nothing should be ruled out.

Q: *Is diabetes difficult to diagnose?*
A: No. The symptoms of insulin-dependent diabetes are marked, making diagnosis easy.

Q: *What are the symptoms?*
A: Excessive passing of urine, thirst, weight loss, lassitude, fatigue.

Q: *My child had those symptoms for a long time before my doctor suggested that it might be diabetes and did a few tests. Why did this happen?*
A: Diabetes in children is not common. Less than 5 percent of persons with diabetes in the United States are under fifteen. And the symptoms of diabetes can also be the symptoms of other, more common, childhood diseases. It is possible that your pediatrician or general practitioner has few if any patients with diabetes.

Q: *Now that my child has been diagnosed, where shall I take him for medical care?*
A: Your family doctor or pediatrician can continue to follow your child for routine testing, immunizations, and minor illnesses. Unless he or she has special training in diabetes, however, you should be referred to a pediatric diabetes specialist or a specialty clinic.

Q: *Where are these specialty clinics located?*
A: Most are located in medical centers or general hospitals, but they may be found in universities, children's hospitals, and private clinics as well. Naturally, in a country as large as ours, there are local variations in care and practice. Your doctor is the best person to advise you.

Q: *What can these specialist clinics offer my child that our pediatrician cannot?*
A: The diabetic clinic will, undoubtedly, be staffed by one or

more endocrinologists or diabetologists, specialists who have an interest and expertise in diabetes. They will have the experience of treating hundreds, perhaps thousands, of people with diabetes. They will have access to the latest equipment. They will have books and magazines about diabetes for you to read. Some clinics have videos and computer programs as well. The diabetic clinic is a place of learning for you and your child. Its educational facilities will probably include a diabetes educator, a health-care professional whose job is to see that every child with diabetes and his family learn about the disease and how to keep it under the best possible control. There will be a dietician to help with meal plans, specialist nurses, perhaps a psychiatrist or therapist, and even a podiatrist.

The clinic may have laboratory facilities and be connected to eye, heart, nerve, and kidney units to detect and treat possible complications before they become severe. Many clinics maintain close links with affiliate groups of national diabetes organizations. These groups provide much assistance, especially in the early days after diagnosis when everything appears so difficult and depressing.

Q: *Do these specialist clinics treat people of all ages, or are there pediatric ones?*

A: It depends on your locality. Some specialist clinics treat adults as well as children, but larger, urban centers generally have diabetic units in their children's hospitals staffed by pediatric endocrinologists. If you have a choice, opt for such a unit. Look for a place where the emphasis is on reassurance and where everything possible is done to make medical care as pleasant as possible for your child. The waiting rooms should be filled with toys and books, the staff should be welcoming and friendly, care should be taken to minimize painful or frightening procedures, and active support should be available to worried parents.

The ideal facility should offer an anesthetic cream for rubbing on small arms before taking blood. The nurses should be pleasant and smiling, prepared to cuddle a whimpering child, and the doctors should be happy to spend as much time as needed to explain matters to anxious parents. Physicians should listen to the parents' ideas even when they aren't perfectly expressed, and he should be willing to follow up any unusual complaint. Thoroughness and interest are characteristics of the good diabetes physician. Going to the doctor is never an experience to which one looks forward eagerly, but the staff should endeavor to create an atmosphere of warmth as well as competence for the child and his parents.

Q: *If I take my child to a specialist clinic, will my family doctor or pediatrician be kept informed of his progress?*
A: It is up to you to request this. You should make clear from the first visit that such communication is necessary and ask that information be sent to your own doctor on a regular basis. It is in your own interest to do so, for specialist clinics are not available on a twenty-four-hour basis, and should your child develop a sudden illness, it will be your own doctor who will be called upon for care. If you lose contact with him, you might find yourself rushing to the emergency room of the children's hospital with every sniffle.

Prepare thoroughly for your visits to the specialist clinic. Produce a detailed medical history and the dates of all his inoculations at the first interview. For your regular three-month visits, write down all the questions you want to ask. Bring his test results. Make the most of your specialist's time and expertise by organizing yourself.

Q: *My family doctor looks after elderly people who have diabetes. Why don't they attend a specialist diabetic clinic?*
A: Some do, of course, but diabetes in the middle-aged and elderly is common in the United States. The internist or physician in general practice probably has many such patients and is experienced in their care.

Q: *I have several elderly relatives who have diabetes. Could my child have inherited the diabetes from them?*
A: It is unlikely that your child's diabetes was inherited directly from these relatives. Diabetes in this older age group is called adult-onset diabetes, Type 2, or non–insulin-dependent diabetes. It is different from the diabetes that your child has developed, which is called juvenile-onset diabetes, Type 1, or insulin-dependent diabetes.

Q: *What is the difference?*
A: In Type 2 diabetes, the pancreas produces insulin, but the cells either cannot take it up and store it or else they cannot release it. Either way, glucose accumulates in the bloodstream. Weight loss, exercise, and medication to lower the blood sugar is usually prescribed to correct the condition. Sometimes insulin by injection is required, but more often it is not. The pancreas can sometimes be stimulated chemically to produce even more insulin. Special diets leading to better weight control are often effective in Type 2 diabetes.

Q: *If my child were to be put on a special diet, would his pancreas be able to make more insulin?*
A: Even on a special diet, his natural insulin would not be sufficient.

Q: *What about stimulating the pancreas chemically? Does this mean taking medication by mouth?*
A: It does, but such treatment is insufficient for Type 1 diabetes, which is always insulin-dependent. Your child's pancreas is unable to produce sufficient quantities of natural insulin because it has too few beta cells. The small amount of insulin that he is producing at the time of diagnosis will be reduced further after a while. He needs insulin injections to supplement his inadequate supply.

Q: *Why can't insulin be given by mouth?*
A: The digestive system would destroy it before it could be used.

Q: *Couldn't the pill be coated with something that the body won't destroy?*
A: This is a possibility for the future, but at present, no one has been able to make such a pill. There is, however, a great deal of research going on all the time in many countries all over the world. Better products will undoubtedly be available in the future. A suitable pill or even a cure could lie around the corner.

Q: *Is diabetes a dangerous disease?*
A: Once the condition is diagnosed and insulin therapy begun, the diabetes can be brought under better control. It can do hidden damage, though. This hidden damage can lead to other diseases in later life that are serious. Abnormal amounts of glucose in the bloodstream interfere with the development of healthy blood vessels, causing them to leak. It allows the buildup of certain fatty acids in the blood, leading to high cholesterol levels. The result could be heart, kidney, eye, and nerve disease, and poor circulation in the extremities. With good control of the blood glucose, however, the likelihood of your child's developing any of these complications in later life is reduced. That is why your knowledge of diabetes is so important.

Q: *Will the diabetes get worse as he gets older?*
A: In the beginning, his body is still producing some insulin. As soon as treatment begins, the pancreas may recover somewhat and insulin production may increase. The amount that has to be added by injection is small, so small that you may begin to wonder if the doctor has made a mistake, that perhaps your child does not have diabetes after all. But after a time, more beta cells will die and the amount of natural insulin will diminish further. He will need more by injection. The early period when the pancreas is still functioning fairly well is called the "honeymoon period."

Q: *How long does the honeymoon period last?*
A: It varies from a few months to a year or more. There is some evidence to suggest that the honeymoon period can be prolonged by good control from the beginning, and this is a worthwhile goal.

Q: *If insulin production is improved during the honeymoon period, will a child be able to stop his injections?*
A: It is rare that enough pancreatic function returns for injections to stop altogether. In fact, many doctors advise continuing with one small injection a day even if insulin needs drop enormously, because they know that in the future, insulin will have to be increased and it may be harder for the child to accept them if injections ceased during the honeymoon period.

Q: *How can I learn more about diabetes?*
A: Read all you can on the subject. A short reading list is given at the end of this book, but many more books about diabetes are available in the public library and in bookstores. Both the Juvenile Diabetes Foundation and the American Diabetes Association (see addresses in the index) publish excellent magazines, books, and pamphlets. They also produce films and videos. You can join these organizations, which have affiliates in every state.

Subscribing to the magazines *Countdown* (JDF) and *Diabetes Forecast* (ADA) will give you much valuable information about diabetes and make certain that you keep up to date with new product development and research. Both magazines contain articles about diabetes care, letters from readers, stories, games and puzzles for children, information about food, and lots of delicious recipes. Another interesting publication is *Health-O-Gram* from the Sugar-free Center. (See Appendix 6 for address.)

You will benefit in many ways from reading these periodicals. Not only will you learn about diabetes, but you will feel that you are coping, keeping on top of things, making things happen rather than waiting until disaster strikes. You will gain strength from the knowledge that you are not alone. Other people with diabetes and their families have similar problems. Learning how they solved theirs will make yours less difficult.

Q: *How do I subscribe?*
A: You can subscribe to *Countdown,* the quarterly magazine of the JDF, for one year by sending a check for $16 to JDF International, 432 Park Ave. South, New York, NY 10016.

For $20 a year, you can join the ADA. Your subscription includes twelve issues of *Diabetic Forecast,* membership in the ADA affiliate group in your area, and a vote in local elections. Send a check or money order to American Diabetes Association, Membership Processing Center, P.O. Box 2055, Harlan, IA 51593-0238.

Q: *What is the value of joining such a group? Isn't it depressing? What will I gain?*
A: Self-help groups provide a forum for learning about diabetes. They arrange meetings with interesting speakers, raise money for diabetes research, and have outings and social events for members, especially children. By joining others to achieve a common goal, many people find that they are better able to cope with stress. The group understands your problems, and this can be a boost to morale. I resisted joining such a group for months after my child was diagnosed and finally joined only to be able to send her to their holiday camp. Once I started attending meetings, however, I was caught up in the group dynamics and soon found myself learning many tips from people with long-standing diabetes. I began reading about diabetes and bringing in interesting bits of information to share with the others at the monthly meetings. Most beneficial of all, when I got involved in the problems of the other members, my own difficulties were easier to bear.

Q: *What can be done if there are no such groups in my town?*
A: Start one yourself. At your specialist clinic or doctor's office, ask for your name to be given to other interested parents. Helping them will help you as well.

Q: *What else do the ADA and JDF do?*
A: Through their many activities, they make life better for those with diabetes. They sponsor research programs to find a cure and lobby for legislation to assist persons with diabetes. They advise on health insurance, product purchase, and medical facilities. They approve centers for diabetes education and ensure that standards are high. Reading their publications will keep you up to date on developments in diet, research, and product development.

Q: *Won't our family physician be aware of new developments in diabetes through the medical journals?*
A: It is unrealistic to expect your general practitioner or even your pediatrician, who may have a small number of children with diabetes in his practice, to keep up completely with research in so specialized a subject.

2

Insulin, Injections, and Reactions

Q: *Where does insulin come from?*
A: Until the last few years, insulin for medical use was made from the pancreas of a cow or pig. Now a synthetic insulin has been developed as well. This synthetic insulin is identical to human insulin. It is free from many impurities, that sometimes provoked allergic reactions in the past.

Q: *How is synthetic human insulin made?*
A: There are two methods for making it at the moment. One is by adjusting porcine (pig) insulin to get it to correspond exactly to natural human insulin. The other method is by changing certain human bacteria into insulin through the use of genetic engineering. This is quite an important advance, because it means that the manufacture of insulin is no longer dependent on the availability of animal pancreases.

Q: *Does this insulin have a special name?*
A: It is called human insulin.

Q: *Is that different from U100?*
A: U100 refers to the strength of the insulin. All insulins used in

the United States, Canada, and Australia are U100. If you travel abroad, it is necessary to check that the insulin available to you is also U100. The insulin used since 1984 in the United Kingdom and Ireland is U100. Some other countries, however, are still using U40 and U80. These have to be given in U40 and U80 syringes, not your usual syringes, which are designed for U100 only.

Q: *Will my child be given animal or human insulin?*
A: Your child's doctor will prescribe the type of insulin that is best for him. All modern insulins are purified, and the results are generally good. Studies of comparative insulins have shown no difference between control on animal and human insulins.

Q: *How should insulin be stored?*
A: It should be kept cool. A refrigerator is best, but make certain that the insulin does not freeze. Don't put it directly under the ice-making compartment, and keep it out of the freezer. When traveling by plane, keep the insulin with you in the cabin of the plane. Do not allow it to be placed in the baggage compartment, where it might be subjected to extremely low temperatures. If you travel by car, buy an insulated insulin container (like a small picnic cooler) or fashion one yourself from polystyrene or even newspapers.

Q: *Should insulin be warmed before injection?*
A: Cold insulin injected into a warm body is uncomfortable. It is better to warm it slightly before use. If you are using a bottle straight from the refrigerator, warm it by rubbing it between your hands for a minute or two before filling the syringe. Although refrigeration is recommended, most people with diabetes store extra bottles of insulin in the refrigerator but keep the bottle or bottles in current use at room temperature. I have never heard of any problems that resulted from this practice.

Q: *My child was prescribed two different kinds of insulin, one clear and one cloudy. What is the difference between them?*
A: The clear insulin is usually referred to as Regular. It is a

quick-acting variety. The cloudy insulin is a long-acting variety called NPH or lente. The cloudy appearance is due to the addition of certain chemicals to slow down its action.

Q: *Why does he need two kinds?*
A: Regular insulin is to provide cover for the meal that comes soon after the shot. NPH or lente is used for meals that will come several hours later. Insulin is required over a twenty-four-hour period. A mixture of Regular and NPH/lente helps to reproduce the body's natural insulin-release pattern.

Q: *How soon after injection does the insulin begin to work?*
A: Regular starts to lower the blood glucose in fifteen to thirty minutes. It continues to work for approximately three to four hours. Regular insulin injected at 7:30 A.M. will start working at breakfast time (assuming that this is 8 A.M.). It will still be active by lunchtime, but will be ineffective by 4 P.M.

NPH and lente insulin works more slowly. It has its strongest effect about eight to fourteen hours after injection. NPH/lente insulin taken at 7:30 A.M. will be active by suppertime but will run out by 9 P.M.

NPH/lente taken before supper (6 P.M.) will cover breakfast the next morning.

Q: *Why are some children on one injection a day, and some on two?*
A: Young children who go to bed at 6 or 7 P.M. can often be adequately controlled on a single injection of Regular and NPH/lente mixed together given in the morning. Regular insulin covers breakfast, midmorning snack, lunch, and afternoon snack. NPH/lente takes care of supper and a bedtime snack. Also, it is likely that the young child, having recently developed diabetes, is still making some natural insulin. Only a small amount of injected insulin is necessary for normal health and growth.

Some children, however, are started on two injections daily right from the beginning no matter how small their insulin needs are. Some doctors think that since most children with diabetes will have to change to two injections eventually, it is easier to begin this routine in the early years.

Q: *Which is better, a one-injection routine or a two?*
A: There are advantages and disadvantages to both. One obvious advantage to a one-injection routine is that injections always appear to be the biggest problem in the beginning and this routine reduces the number by half. A disadvantage is that the child is tied to an early supper. On a one-injection routine, he must have his supper when the NPH/lente is at its peak action. If his shot was at 7:30 in the morning, he must eat his evening meal by 5 o'clock or his blood glucose will drop too low. While a three-year-old is happy to eat at that hour, a school-age child may want to be out playing with his friends at 5 o'clock.

Naturally, if your doctor recommends a particular routine, you should follow his advice. Some children have more natural insulin production than others in the early days after diagnosis, and your doctor's choice of routine will be influenced by that factor as well as others. If your child is put on a two-injection schedule from the beginning, you can console yourself (and the child) with the thought that eventually he would have to change to that routine anyway, and that the two-injection regime allows more latitude.

Q: *If my child is on two shots a day, can supper be eaten at any time?*
A: It is important to stick to a fairly regular timetable for meals and shots to ensure that the insulin in circulation is the right amount at the time. You need to be certain that meals are taken when the insulin is at its peak action so that blood glucose does not fall below normal. It is possible, however, to be more flexible on a two-injection routine, moving the evening mealtime to 6 P.M. or even 7 P.M. without problems. On a two-injection routine, the morning dose of NPH/lente is smaller than it would be on a single-dose schedule. The afternoon snack can be taken after school, allowing more freedom in the early evening for play before sup-

per. In fact, if your child has been on a single-injection routine and has to change to two injections a day, this can be a convincing argument. If he were willing to take two injections, he would not be tied to an early-evening meal and would be spared the risk of low blood glucose around 5 o'clock, when he might want to be playing ball or riding his bike. My child resisted changing to two injections until she became a member of the swimming team and had to practice from 4 to 5 every day. At ten years old (and two years with diabetes), she decided that the risk of an insulin reaction at the swimming pool was much worse than an extra shot.

Q: *You say that injections appear to be the biggest problem at first. Do they get easier after a while?*
A: It is hard to believe when your child is first diagnosed, but injections really do get easier after a while. In a year or two, injections will become almost automatic. Your child will hardly mind them as much as brushing his teeth. I know that statement sounds unbelievable to the parent of a newly diagnosed child, but it really is true. After a while, the child will become completely casual about injections and regard anyone who balks at them as foolish. (I don't guarantee, however, that the parents will feel the same way!)

Q: *If my child has to take both Regular and NPH/lente once or twice a day, does this mean that he has to take two injections each time, or can the two types be mixed in the same syringe?*
A: Check this point with your doctor, but most people mix insulins. You do it in the following way:

1. Wash your hands.
2. Clean the tops of the bottles with alcohol on a piece of cotton or with an alcohol swab.
3. Shake the bottle of NPH/lente to ensure that it is evenly mixed. (If you cannot get it to mix evenly, discard it and use another bottle. Return it to your druggist if it retains bits that won't dissolve.)

4. With your syringe, inject air into the NPH/lente in an amount corresponding to the prescribed units of insulin. (If you need to draw up 10 units of insulin, inject 10 units of air.)
5. Withdraw the syringe. Do not draw up any insulin yet.
6. Insert the same syringe into the Regular insulin. Inject the required units of air. (If you need to draw up 15 units of insulin, inject 15 units of air.)
7. Do not remove the syringe. Draw up the Regular insulin.
8. Return to the NPH/lente bottle. Draw up the insulin.
9. Tap out any bubbles of air that may have appeared in the syringe.
10. If recommended by your doctor, swab the injection site with alcohol and inject.

Q: *Why is it necessary to clean the top of the bottles with alcohol?*
A: I recommend cleaning the bottle tops only because it is likely that your child will keep his diabetic kit in a plastic box that will soon become a repository for crumbs, used syringes, old plastic testing strips, notebooks, pencils, etc. It will probably make you feel better to introduce a hygienic note. However, if you run out of alcohol swabs, don't panic. It is extremely unlikely that bacteria will find their way from the top of the insulin bottle into the syringe.

Q: *I have seen older people with diabetes take their shots without swabbing the site. Is it necessary?*
A: I have heard of a doctor with diabetes who injects through his trouser leg and has never had an infection. I should not recommend that you try it, however. Check with your physician on this point. There are two schools of opinion. If you do swab, though, be prepared for the sight of a few skin cells coming off on the cotton. People with white skin will hardly see them, but black people will.

Q: *What do you do if, in the middle of filling the syringe, you find that you have made a mistake?*
A: Discard the insulin and start again. Soon you and your child will become expert and mistakes will be rare. In the beginning, everyone is clumsy and uncertain about shots. We all recoil from the needle. Expertise, however, is quickly acquired. Before long, you will be helping someone new.

Q: *Is there any way that I can make shots less painful for my child? He gets upset each time. This is upsetting to me, too.*
A: Try putting an ice cube on the site for a short time to make the skin less sensitive. He will probably think it is fun. In fact, many children like to suck ice cubes, and you could let him do that to distract him from the actual shot after you have chilled the site.

Much of the unpleasantness associated with injections is psychological. The prick of the needle is almost painless if the needle is sharp and fine. Most needles on the market today are lubricated for greater comfort. The "pain" is mostly fear, his and yours. Children sense fear much as animals do. If you present a calm and reassuring front to your child at shot time, it will help him to relax. If this is difficult for you, you might find that someone else, perhaps an older child, can help. It does not always have to be Mommy or Daddy who do these things. Don't feel that you have failed if you withdraw in favor of Grandma or Sister or a friend. A child who is newly diagnosed can present many problems. It often takes the resources of many people to cope. Just keep telling yourself that this trying time will not last forever.

Q: *Is injection the only way of taking insulin?*
A: At the moment, it is the way in general use. Research is going on every day, however, to find better methods of insulin delivery. There are even experiments in inhaling insulin through the nose and taking it rectally in a suppository. I doubt that either of these two methods will be used widely, however. But one new delivery system that was extremely popular a few years ago is the insulin pump. This is a device worn outside the body on a belt at the waist

or in a shoulder holster. The pump contains a small reservoir of insulin connected to a plastic tube. A fine needle, attached to the other end of the tube, is inserted under the skin, usually into the abdomen, and taped in place. There is even a pump with a non-needle infuser, which is virtually painless. The pumps are powered by rechargeable batteries and hold up to 300 units of U100 insulin. The newer ones have a built-in alarm to give warning in the event of a problem.

The pump releases a small quantity of insulin at a continuous rate throughout the day. This is called the basal rate. Whenever the wearer wishes to eat a meal, he can release a larger dose, called a bolus. The pump, then, mimics the body's own natural insulin action and provides excellent control for the wearer provided that care is taken to operate it perfectly.

Q: *Are these pumps suitable for children?*

A: Pumps are very exciting, and most parents see them as a way to get away from shots. They are not, however, the answer for everyone. Although the smallest pump is the size of a plastic credit card, most are quite a bit larger. The needle site must be changed every 48 to 72 hours hours to avoid infection. To ensure that the pump is working properly and to calculate how large the bolus of insulin should be before a meal, the wearer must test his blood five or six times a day. Many children find this irksome. A school-age child would have to find a time and place to do his tests under difficult conditions, and the preschooler would not like to be called in from play continually to have his finger pricked. The pump has to be removed for swimming and bathing, and care must be exercised so that air does not get into the tubing when it is reattached. Another problem is that the pump is filled only with Regular insulin. If there is a delivery failure, hyperglycemia (high blood glucose) could develop very rapidly and could even progress to ketoacidosis before anyone realizes what has happened. It is also very expensive, although many health-insurance policies will cover part of the cost. Still, for all its drawbacks, the pump has great advantages. It allows the careful wearer to achieve near-normal blood glucose values. As such, it is excellent for use under special conditions like pregnancy or by people who are willing to spend the time and money to look after their diabetes exceedingly well. It is worthwhile considering a pump for an older child or teenager if you and your doctor think that the child has the commitment necessary to make it work.

Q: *Have you any experience with children wearing a pump?*
A: I was involved in a pump study several years ago in which twenty children were given a pump and monitored carefully. Half did very well, achieving excellent control. The other half gave up the pump for various reasons before the study was completed.

Q: *What were the problems?*
A: Several of the girls balked at the restrictions on dress. It was necessary to wear this particular pump on a belt at the waist, which meant that only skirts and blouses could be worn unless the wearer was prepared to cut a hole in the dress. One sixteen-year-old girl said she found it embarrassing to be attached to something when necking with her boyfriend.

Some of the children suffered from diabetic ketoacidosis (extremely high blood glucose with ketones) due to pump failure, generally a clogged needle. They required hospitalization. These incidents frightened both children and parents, and the affected children returned to conventional insulin therapy. This study took place several years ago, however; pumps are now lighter, less bulky, and have needles that are less likely to clog. There are also implantable pumps.

Q: *What are implantable pumps?*
A: These are similar in concept to a cardiac pacemaker. They are implanted under the skin of the abdomen and operated by means of a radio signal like those that open the garage door or turn the channel on the television set. The pumps have a reservoir of insulin whose basal and bolus rates can be set and changed by means of these signals. The reservoirs can be topped up by a

hypodermic needle when necessary. Pumps eliminate the problem of inserting a needle under the skin and changing the site frequently. And, of course, they are invisible. They may have other problems, though, such as blockage and interference with the signals. They are also extremely expensive but should, if their use becomes more widespread, be reduced in price. Naturally, they have to be inserted under an anesthetic in the hospital. That is a simple procedure, however. They also need close monitoring, and this means a big commitment on the part of both the wearer and the members of the health-care team.

Q: *Would you recommend a pump for children?*
A: Pump therapy is new. I think that parents should wait until research and development is more advanced. It is hoped that the pump, especially the implantable pump, will eventually be able to be linked to a blood-glucose sensor, which would test the glucose levels and automatically release the correct amount of insulin. This would be virtually an artificial pancreas. If such a device could be developed, it would revolutionize the treatment of diabetes.

Q: *Is it likely that such a device will be developed?*
A: Much work is being done in this country and abroad to develop it. With the gigantic advances in biotechnology in the last few years, I think that we may well see a breakthrough. Animal models are crucial to this work. Insulin was originally isolated by use of experiments on dogs. Human tissue is needed, too, so think carefully before you take sides in moves to limit medical research and experimentation with animal or human tissue.

Q: *Are any people with diabetes in the United States wearing pumps at the moment?*
A: Yes. Many are wearing them, and the number will increase in the future. Pumps are becoming better, smaller, less expensive, and freer from problems every day. It is still too early, however, to know whether the pump is the answer for everyone.

Q: *Are any of these pump users children?*
A: Yes, some of them are. If you would like to talk to someone who is wearing a pump or who is the parent of a child wearing a pump, your diabetic doctor should be able to arrange it.

Q: *Are there any other new devices that are suitable for children?*
A: One interesting device is the infuser button. It is a flat plastic device the size and shape of a small coin. A fine needle is inserted into the abdomen and taped into place, connecting the button to the body. At shot time, the wearer injects into the button. The shot, therefore, is painless. It enables the user to inject many times during the day rather than once or twice. He can take a small dose of Regular insulin whenever he eats, mimicking more closely the release of natural insulin. He would need, however, to have a shot of very-long-acting insulin once a day to release a small amount of insulin over a twenty-four-hour period to provide a base. For the conscientious user, the button can mean better control.

Q: *Would you recommend the infuser button for children?*
A: It might be suitable for the older child. To get the maximum advantage from the button, frequent blood tests would have to be done. Also, the button itself would have to be moved every forty-eight hours (perhaps even more frequently) to avoid infection at the site. The manufacturers recommend moving it every three days, but individual reactions vary and some people might require a more frequent move. Although it is certainly an interesting idea, and one that is inexpensive, your own doctor is the best person to consult. He or she will know whether it is suitable for your child.

Q: *Are there any ways of taking insulin that don't require a needle?*
A: There are several needle-free injectors on the market. These devices work by shooting a fine stream of insulin, about one third the size of the finest needle, at the skin at such high velocity that it penetrates from its own force. It has been developed from

injection guns used in the armed forces to inoculate thousands of men in a very short time. Your doctor will be able to advise you about their use. There have been problems in the past with damage to the tissue and about dispersal of the insulin. The manufacturers have been trying to overcome these problems, and if they succeed, it might be a good solution for a child who is frightened of injections. Still, it is a more cumbersome device than a syringe and is quite expensive.

Q: *I have seen advertisements for an insulin pen. What is that?*
A: The insulin pen is proving to be the most popular of the newer delivery systems and one that has much to recommend it. The device looks like an ordinary fountain pen and like a pen is filled with a cartridge, not of ink, but of Regular insulin. The user takes one shot of a very-long-acting insulin once a day, usually in the evening although it can be at any time that suits him, for base-rate insulin function. Then he injects Regular insulin with the pen whenever he has a meal. This means that the average person takes four shots a day. The needle in the pen is extremely fine and shots are virtually painless. The pen can be set to deliver a prearranged dose very quickly and discreetly, and it is this element of discretion that has made the pen so popular with teenagers and adults alike. It allows freedom from preset mealtimes and prearranged portions because each meal is covered separately. Most of its users do not find the extra shots a problem, but like all these devices, the price of better control is extra vigilance. Frequent blood-glucose tests are necessary to determine insulin amounts.

Q: *Would you recommend the pen?*
A: Again, I think it is an excellent delivery system for the older child who is highly motivated and experienced in managing his condition. My own teenage daughter has one and loves it. She has found that she is off the hook of rigid schedules and can indulge in a late-night hamburger with her friends without worry that it will increase her blood glucose. She just takes a few extra units with the pen. It is part of the new intensive therapy that uses frequent

glucose tests to adjust the insulin dose before every meal. For the newly diagnosed child, however, intensive therapy is probably not required or desirable. Your doctor will know exactly which delivery system is best for your child. Even if he wants the child to use a pen after the honeymoon period, you and your youngster should master the basic technique of giving shots first. Diabetes is for life, and you never know when such skills will be needed.

Q: *Since my child has to have shots, how can I get him to accept them more easily?*
A: The young child has already established a pattern of accepting whatever his parents present to him. If the parents have a matter-of-fact attitude toward his injections, he will learn very quickly to accept them. With an older child, it might take longer, but in my experience as a diabetes educator for many years, children accept shots more readily than their parents would have believed possible. Sometimes play can help. I know one nine-year-old who played "hospital" constantly after she was diagnosed. By injecting dolls and stuffed animals, she was able to work through her anger at developing diabetes. Play like this can be a useful tool and should not be discouraged even if it appears morbid to outsiders. Sometimes, though, injection aids can be used to get the child over the hump.

Q: *What are injection aids?*
A: These are devices that are designed to assist in getting the needle into the body quickly and at the right angle for the most efficient absorption of insulin. They fit over the end of the syringe, hiding the needle from view. The user places the device against the skin and exerts a little pressure. The needle shoots in quickly and the plunger is then pushed manually. In some injectors, the plunger is automatic too. It makes the shot easier for many children and for those adults who are squeamish about needles. It made life in our house much more pleasant when we were presented with an injection aid by a more experienced parent when our child was first diagnosed.

Q: *Where can I get such a device?*
A: They are advertised in the diabetes magazines and in mail-order catalogues. They are available in shops like the Sugar-free Center in California (see address in Appendix 6) and in some drugstores.

Q: *Are they expensive?*
A: Considering the comfort that a child receives from the device, I think that they are very reasonable. It is possible that your medical insurance will cover it. Check your policy details.

Q: *Does the aid have to be sterilized before using?*
A: Instructions for keeping the aid will be in the box. Generally, it is kept in a plastic container filled with denatured alcohol.

Q: *Are there any drawbacks to these aids?*
A: The biggest disadvantage is that the child becomes dependent on the aid and will not inject without it. This could be a problem if the gadget is lost or damaged. I think that if a child is not unduly frightened by injections, it is better to learn good injection technique from the beginning. If injections are a trial, however, if tears and fussing are a daily ritual, an injection aid might solve the problem.

Q: *What constitutes good injection technique?*
A: The syringe must be filled correctly (see page 33) and any air bubbles tapped out. A suitable site must be selected (see illustration in Appendix 1) and the child should sit comfortably with his feet on the floor. He should then inject straight in at a right angle to the skin.

Q: *The nurse in the hospital showed us how to inject. She said to inject at an angle of 45 degrees. Which is correct?*
A: If you are using the newest, finest needle available (which is the one that will cause the least discomfort), you will find that this needle is only ½ inch or ⅝ of an inch long. The nurse was

probably trained at a time when needles for insulin shots were much longer. If you inject at an angle of forty-five degrees with a short needle, you will get a shallow injection that will leave insulin in a mass under the skin because it hasn't reached the subcutaneous layer of fat that lies underneath. Absorption will be poor and irregular and control will suffer. Why not get a new insulin syringe and show it to the nurse? Perhaps she will change her advice.

Q: *I didn't know that there were syringes with needles of various lengths. Which is the best?*
A: The shortest, finest needles are the most comfortable to use. At the moment, that is a 29-gauge needle lubricated to give an easier shot. The figure 29 refers to the width of the needle. The finer the needle, the higher the gauge. Look for the shortest needle with the highest gauge number.

Q: *Where can I get syringes with such fine needles?*
A: They are probably available at your local drugstore. If not, there are several mail-order houses that sell diabetes supplies. Advertisements for these appear in the diabetes magazines. If you do not subscribe to these magazines yet, your doctor's office may have back copies. Ask the nurse.

Q: *I have seen syringes with the needles attached and some with the needles separate. Which are the best?*
A: Many people prefer the syringes with the needles permanently attached, because there is no danger of the needle's coming off during the shot, which can be upsetting, especially to a child. There is very little between them, however. It is slightly more economical to use the syringe with the detachable needles, because you can change the needle while re-using the syringe.

Q: *Is it possible to re-use the disposable syringe? The packet warns you to throw them away after one use.*
A: Recent medical surveys in Great Britain have found no evidence of infection due to the re-use of plastic syringes, and most

doctors there advise their patients to use them until the needle is blunt. In the United States, attitudes are more cautious. Whether this is due to medical convention or to the high incidence of lawsuits, I do not know. Your own doctor is the best person to advise you about the re-use of disposable syringes. My child uses them until she feels that they are no longer at their peak of sharpness.

Q: *Is it necessary to sterilize needles if you re-use them?*
A: Sterilizing a plastic syringe is not recommended. If you boiled it, it would disintegrate; if you wiped it with alcohol, the numbers would rub off and, after a few times, it would fall apart. If your physician agrees that you can re-use them, just replace the plastic cap that fits over the needle. Slide it down carefully so that the needle never comes in contact with the plastic (to avoid blunting it), then store it in a convenient place. A glass or jar on the door of the refrigerator is a handy place. It may be kept anywhere, though. My child used to keep all her gear in a plastic storage box and an extra set in a handbag for traveling. If she went out for a meal straight after school, she just took her little bag with her in the morning and didn't have the bother of transferring bottles and syringes from the box. If your child has a friend with whom he stays for supper or sleeps over, you might want to keep an extra set at the friend's house.

Q: *How do you dispose of used syringes?*
A: Put them into containers. Don't throw them into the trash. If possible, cut the needles off as well. Be especially careful these days, with the drug culture so pervasive. Don't leave needles or syringes in a place where an addict could get hold of them.

Q: *Will my child always have to have injections?*
A: If he has insulin-dependent diabetes, he will always have to have insulin. At the moment, the only insulin delivery system in general use is injection.

Q: *Are two shots a day the most he will ever need?*
A: Multiple-injection therapy has become popular in the last few years. This intensive treatment has proved to be more effective in keeping blood-glucose levels normal than one or two injections. If your child has just been diagnosed, however, he is still in the honeymoon period and making some natural insulin, and he probably does not require intensive therapy. Your doctor is the best judge. However, there may be times, especially during illness or unexplained periods of high blood-glucose levels, when an extra shot is required. However incredible it may seem to you now, extra shots will cease to be a problem after a while and you will easily suggest to your child that he take a bit of extra insulin when required.

Q: *Who should do the injections?*
A: Ideally, the patient himself with diabetes should do them. If the child is very young, of course, the parent has to do them for him.

Q: *At what age should the child do his own?*
A: This varies with the ability and attitude of the child and his parents. I know children of six who do their own shots and are quite proud of their independence. I also know children many years older who refuse to do them or whose parents won't allow them to take on this responsibility. I think that you should regard this in the same way that you regard other aspects of growing up. As soon as the child is able to take over, he should be encouraged to do so. If you are looking for a simple answer, I think that eight years old is a reasonable age to expect this kind of independence, although even then, responsibility will be shared, and the parent should not be disappointed if a child agrees to inject himself some of the time but still expects the parent to administer many of the shots. Growing up is rarely simple, and the ball is often bounced from the parental court to the child's and back again many times before the matter is settled.

Q: *Should a young child be allowed to fill the syringe?*
A: It is better to supervise this aspect of care for a few more years until you are confident that your child can manage it without error. You will find that he will become quite expert in giving his shots in a very short time.

Q: *Is it more painful to take a long time to administer the shot or to do it quickly? My child accepted shots while in the hospital when they were given by the nurses, but cries when I do them. I am inexperienced, of course, and slow.*
A: The least painful shot is the one given most quickly. The nerve endings are in the skin. The quicker the layers of skin are penetrated, the less the pain is felt.

Q: *How can I increase my speed?*
A: Speed will come automatically with experience. Have you ever watched a master chef on TV cutting an onion? How deftly he dissects it into hundreds of tiny, even pieces! It takes years of practice, though, to develop this quick, apparently careless ease. It might help you to practice with a chicken. Next time you cook a chicken, try piercing its flesh with an insulin syringe. Note how much easier it is to get through the skin quickly if you hold the chicken firmly and toss the needle in like a dart.

Q: *What do you do about air bubbles in the syringe? I am terrified about injecting air into a vein and killing my child.*
A: This is one of the most common fears about giving shots to oneself or anyone else. If you look closely at an insulin syringe, though, you will notice that it is quite narrow and that the needle is short. The places where you are injecting insulin have layers of fat under the skin. The short needle cannot reach the large blood vessels. It can go only into the fat layers. Also, if you examine the air bubbles that appear in the syringe, they are tiny. There isn't room for large bubbles of air inside such a narrow space. Such small quantities of air will not do any harm.

Still, you should try to get rid of the bubbles so that you take all your insulin by flicking the syringe with your finger. If you cannot, turn it upside down after it is filled. Wait until the contents settle and turn it up again. You will find that the insulin has returned to the front of the syringe, leaving the air bubbles behind. Inject before the bubbles make their way back.

Q: *What do you do if some insulin oozes out again?*
A: This is bound to happen occasionally. Just pull the skin to one side, closing off the puncture. Next time you inject, pull the skin aside before injection. As soon as the syringe is empty and the needle withdrawn, return the skin to its original position, thus closing the hole and preventing leakage.

Q: *Should there be a little lump under the skin after injection?*
A: No. If you are getting a lump, the shot is too shallow. Make certain that you are putting the needle straight down at a right angle to the skin.

Q: *Why is there sometimes a small amount of bleeding?*
A: You have probably pierced a very small blood vessel called a capillary. This is nothing to worry about. The bleeding stops in a few seconds. It may discolor the skin for a few days. This happens to everyone sometimes, but it is not a frequent occurrence. Don't worry about it.

Q: *Is there a problem of injecting into a large blood vessel?*
A: If you use the sites recommended by your doctor (see illustration in Appendix 1), there is no danger. These sites have been chosen because they do not contain major blood vessels or nerves.

Q: *How important is it to vary the sites? My child is resistant to the idea of injecting anywhere but one small area of the leg.*
A: Quite important. If one site were used repeatedly, the tissue

would become hard and insulin absorption irregular. Control would suffer. Other problems might arise as a result. The favorite site might become pain-resistant, which would make the child favor it more. Avoid this problem from the beginning. It can lead to trouble. Make sure that your child understands the reason for changing the sites. If he is young, perhaps you could make a chart together to hang in his room showing the correct sites and labeling them "Monday," "Tuesday," etc. You could enlarge the illustration in Appendix 1. If he is willing to inject into his stomach as well as the legs (arms are usually too small in young children), let him do his morning injection into his tummy and the evening one into his leg, or vice versa. This sort of regularity gives the best results because the insulin is absorbed at the same rate at the same time every day. The first principle of good control is *regularity.*

Q: *Are there other factors that affect the rate of absorption of insulin?*
A: Insulin is most quickly absorbed from the abdomen, then the arms, followed by the thighs and buttocks. Heat and activity affect it as well. Heat causes insulin to circulate more rapidly through the bloodstream. If a shot is followed by a hot bath or a long, hot shower, the circulation is speeded up and blood-glucose levels are lowered quickly.

If vigorous exercise like biking follows a shot into the legs or thighs, the insulin circulates more quickly than if the child is sitting quietly watching television. This characteristic of insulin can be used to increase control. For example, if a finger prick before a shot indicates that the blood glucose is slightly higher than normal, an alternative to increasing the Regular insulin and running the risk of an insulin reaction a few hours later is to reduce the glucose levels by speeding up the circulation.

Q: *Can the circulation be speeded up in any other way?*
A: You could rub the spot gently for five minutes, raising the skin temperature by friction, or you could warm it by placing a hot water bottle wrapped in a towel or a heating pad on the site. Be

very careful that the temperature is not hot, only comfortably warm.

Q: *Should parents insist that injection sites be varied?*
A: Suggestion is better than insistence. A tactful way to get your child to vary the sites is to send him to one of the children's diabetes camps run by the various diabetes organizations. There he will see other children injecting into their arms and tummies as well as their legs. He will want to try it too. Children are natural conformists. They are happiest doing what other children do. It gives them a sense of belonging. These camps are extremely valuable for the child who is newly diagnosed. Your child can enjoy himself in perfect security and learn about his diabetes at the same time. The camps also give parents some time off from the responsibility of caring for a child with special needs, which can be very difficult at first.

Q: *What kinds of activities do they have at camp?*
A: There are all the usual vacation activities such as swimming, hiking, perhaps biking or horseback riding, canoeing, arts and crafts, sports like tennis and baseball, discos, etc. The children are looked after by trained counselors, many of them older teenagers or young adults who have diabetes themselves. Doctors and nurses are plentiful and meals are planned by qualified dieticians. Camp is generally a wonderful experience for the child with diabetes, who finds that he is no different from the others and can relax, let down his guard, and have fun.

Q: *Are these camps expensive?*
A: If cost is your worry, contact your nearest affiliate and explain your problem. Diabetes self-help groups raise money for research and to assist families with diabetes. It is most likely that a way will be found to reduce the cost of camp for you.

Q: *Where are these camps located?*
A: Write to the American Diabetes Association (address in Ap-

pendix 6) to find the camp nearest to your home. Next to choosing a sympathetic doctor in whom you have confidence, you will probably find it the most worthwhile step you can take in coping with the problem of the newly diagnosed child.

Q: *I have heard a lot about insulin reactions. What exactly happens in an insulin reaction and is this the same as hypoglycemia?*
A: An insulin reaction is caused by hypoglycemia, which just means low blood glucose. Although the scientific definition of hypoglycemia is a blood glucose lower than 40 milligrams per deciliter (mg/dl), it is possible to show symptoms at levels higher than this, and I have known small children to tolerate even lower levels. At whatever level your child shows symptoms of an insulin reaction, though, these symptoms should never be ignored.

Q: *What are the symptoms?*
A: Weakness, sweating, trembling, irritability, blurred vision, numbness around the mouth, headache, stomachache, confusion, acting drunk, possibly vomiting. Everyone won't get all these symptoms every time, but you should suspect an insulin reaction if even one of these signs is present.

Q: *Does someone with diabetes get a warning when a reaction is coming on?*
A: It varies. I have found that reactions can be divided into two sorts: mild and severe. The severity of the reaction is dependent on how quickly the blood glucose drops. If it drops gradually, he will have warning signs. He may have one or more of the symptoms described above. He may also cry, sulk, be angry, or become unreasonable. If sugar is given as soon as these signs appear, the reaction usually subsides in a few minutes and the child is normal again. If they go unnoticed, of course, the blood glucose will continue to drop and the child could become unconscious. There are some episodes of hypoglycemia that give no warning, however. The person may become unconscious almost immediately. These are rare in childhood. A severe reaction is also rare in the child

who is generally well controlled, but it can happen, probably because the insulin is suddenly being absorbed more quickly than normal. These develop so rapidly that often the blood glucose has dropped to the level where the child is completely unreasonable before anyone realizes what has happened.

Q: *What happens if my child has a reaction in his sleep? Could he become unconscious without anyone's noticing?*
A: Nighttime reactions are every parent's nightmare. Indeed, it is frightening, especially the first one. The early warning stages pass unnoticed in sleep. Then the child awakens, cries, even screams. He may thrash around in his bed and be completely unreasonable and uncontrollable, especially if he is too large to handle. It is difficult to persuade him to eat or drink. If sugar is pushed into his mouth, he may spit it out. Still, it is not likely that he will become unconscious. It is more usual for him to waken and cry.

Q: *If he refuses to take sugar, what can be done?*
A: There are several things that can be done. But don't offer a sweet drink from a glass if he is screaming and throwing himself around the bed. The drink will get everywhere but inside his mouth. Keep a jar of honey or corn syrup handy. Rub some inside his mouth. He will swallow it along with his saliva. Be careful. He might bite you. He will become completely unreasonable and most likely belligerent. If you have a plastic bottle used to wash off testing strips, you can fill it with a sweet drink. These bottles have a curved spout that you can put into his mouth. You might manage to squirt in enough sugar to restore his glucose levels to normal. There are also plastic bottles and tubes of concentrated glucose that you can buy in the drugstore or a mail-order diabetes supply house. This can be put into his mouth if he can be persuaded to suck it. If all else fails, you can resort to glucagon.

Q: *What is glucagon?*
A: Glucagon is a hormone produced in the islets of Langerhans,

just as insulin is. The beta cells make insulin. The alpha cells make glucagon. Its effect is the opposite from that of insulin. Its presence in the bloodstream causes the liver to release some of its stored glucose. Blood-glucose levels rise and the reaction is over.

Q: *How is it used?*
A: It is injected much like insulin. You fill a clean insulin syringe with glucagon and inject it into the thigh. You may have to sit on the child in order to do this. Even with a small child, it often takes two adults to accomplish this unless the child has lost consciousness. In ten to twenty minutes, the child will begin to recover. Then you can give a sweet drink, followed by small amounts of carbohydrate food at frequent intervals. It is likely that he will vomit when his glucose levels rise. Then you will have to get him to take more carbohydrates. When he is nauseous, Coca-Cola allowed to go flat is usually tolerated better than Gatorade or fruit juice.

Q: *What happens if the glucagon doesn't work?*
A: If the child has not recovered within fifteen or twenty minutes of the administration of glucagon, take him immediately to the emergency room of the nearest hospital, or call 911. He probably needs an IV.

Q: *Is glucagon difficult to use?*
A: The difficulty in using glucagon is that you are using it under stressful conditions. It is a good idea to practice with an out-of-date glucagon set for some time so that you will gain confidence. Ask your doctor or diabetes educator for instructions in its use.

Q: *Is it dangerous if too much is administered?*
A: It isn't a drug, merely a hormone. The amount in the bottle is small, so this is not a problem.

Q: *Where can I get glucagon?*
A: From your drugstore on prescription. It is available as a

"glucagon emergency kit" or as "glucagon for injection, USP." The emergency kit is easier to use, because it contains a syringe filled with sterile water and an ampoule of glucagon. The USP preparation must be mixed from a powder and then injected with a regular 1-cc (not low-dose) syringe.

Q: *Do doctors approve of its use by parents?*
A: Some don't. If your doctor doesn't want you to use it, and you cannot get a child in an insulin reaction to take sugar, all you can do is bring him to a hospital.

Q: *What would happen if no one heard his cries?*
A: Possibly, he would go back to sleep and his glucose levels would rise naturally in response to the hypoglycemia. When he awoke in the morning, he would have a headache and perhaps a stomachache too. He might remember a bad dream. Many nighttime reactions do pass unnoticed. The body has a natural mechanism for coping with low glucose levels. As glucose levels fall, the level of glucagon in the body will rise, triggering the release of more glucose from the liver. When you inject glucagon artificially, you are merely speeding up this natural process.

Q: *Why is it necessary to speed it up? It sounds difficult and frightening. Why not just leave it to happen naturally?*
A: It is possible that the lack of glucose in the brain for a prolonged period might cause brain damage. Although rare, this can happen. It is better to take no chances and do whatever one can to increase the glucose levels quickly.

3

Control

Q: *Throughout, you have mentioned good diabetes control, but how can this be measured?*

A: It can be measured by testing the urine and/or blood to determine how much glucose is present. It can also be measured by testing the urine for the presence of ketones or fatty acids.

Q: *Can these tests be performed at home?*

A: Yes. They can and they should.

Q: *Is special equipment necessary?*

A: Yes, but it is easily obtained. Equipment for testing both urine and blood is available in drugstores and through mail-order drug companies.

Q: *How do you test the urine?*

A: It can be tested with reagent tablets and reagent strips. Let's look at the strip method first, as this is the most popular and the simplest.

1. Testing for Glucose by Reagent Strips

Get a bottle of reagent strips at your local drugstore. Tell the druggist that you want strips to test urine for glucose. It is a common request, and he will know what to sell you.

Wet the end of the strip with urine by passing it through the urine stream for two seconds. Boys can do this easily, of course. Girls can do it, too, with a bit of care. If girls find it difficult, however, they can catch the urine in a little basin or jar and dip the strip into it.

Wait for 30 seconds. (Check your package directions. The most popular brand reacts in 30 seconds, but another brand might require more or less time.) Shake the excess urine off the strip. Immediately compare the colored patch on the end of the strip with the color chart on the bottle. The colored square that best matches the test area tells you how much glucose is present in the urine.

2. Testing for Glucose by Reagent Tablets

(A) 5-DROP METHOD

Get a bottle of reagent tablets at the drugstore. The most popular brands come as sets consisting of a bottle of tablets, a chart, a test tube, and a plastic dropper.

Collect the urine in a jar or basin. Fill the dropper and put 5 drops into the test tube. Discard the rest and wash the dropper.

Add 10 drops of water to the test tube.

Put one tablet into the test tube. Do not touch it with your fingers. The easiest way to handle the tablets is to shake one into the bottle's cap and gently tip it into the test tube. Recap the bottle instantly.

Holding the test tube at the top (it will get hot), watch the liquid foam up and change color.

Fifteen seconds after the boiling has stopped, shake the tube gently and compare the color with the chart in the box.

(B) 2-DROP METHOD

This method is sometimes recommended to test higher levels of glucose, especially in small children. If your doctor recommends the two-drop method, you proceed in exactly the same way except that you use 2 drops of urine and 10 drops of water. A special color chart for use with this method is inside the box.

3. Testing for Ketones by Reagent Strips

Get a bottle of strips from the drugstore. The most popular brand is called Ketostix. Your druggist will know what to sell you if you tell him that you want to test urine for ketones.

Wet the strip in the same way as for glucose testing. Wait for 30 seconds or as long as the instructions indicate. "Read" the strip by comparing it to the color chart on the bottle.

4. Testing for Ketones by Reagent Tablets

Get a bottle of reagent tablets from the drugstore. Acetest is a common brand.

Collect the urine in a jar or basin.

Shake one tablet out. Do not touch it with your fingers. Close the bottle at once. With a dropper, place one drop of urine on the tablet. Compare the color changes with the chart in the package. Wash all traces of the tablet down the sink when you are finished.

Q: *What are ketones and why do you have to test for them?*
A: Ketones are fatty acids in the body. If the body is unable to use glucose (because of lack of insulin), it breaks down fat molecules and ketones are released. If the urine shows signs of ketones, it indicates that this process is taking place and that more insulin is required to stop it.

Q: *What is acetone? In the hospital, my child was tested for acetones. Is this the same as ketones?*
A: Acetone is one type of ketone.

Q: *How often should the urine be tested?*
A: Unless you are directed differently by your physician, test once a day for glucose and, if all is well and no glucose is found, once a week for ketones. If glucose is found in the urine, however, it is a good idea to test it for ketones as well. If moderate or large amounts of ketones are present, the doctor should be called. During illness, the urine should be tested for ketones frequently.

Q: *What is a normal reading?*
A: A normal reading shows no glucose or ketones in the urine. This is not an entirely accurate guide to diabetic control, however, because glucose normally does not spill over into the urine until the levels in the blood are quite a bit higher than normal. The absence of glucose in the urine really means that the level of glucose in the bloodstream is below 180 mg/dl, the level at which it first appears in the urine. This level, called the renal threshold, may change in adulthood.

The normal range of glucose in the bloodstream is 72 mg/dl to 126 mg/dl. A negative reading in a urine test, then, indicates only that the blood glucose is less than 180 mg/dl. It cannot tell us whether the blood glucose is slightly elevated—say, between 144 mg/dl and 180 mg/dl—or whether it is below normal and the child is in danger of having a hypoglycemic reaction. Urine testing is a useful tool, especially in illness, but it needs to be supplemented.

Q: *Are there other methods of testing?*
A: Yes. Blood testing gives more information.

Q: *Can blood be tested at home?*
A: Yes. The single most important advance in the control of diabetes since the discovery of insulin in 1921 is self-monitoring of blood glucose. The technique is simple, and with it the person with diabetes can alter his insulin, diet, and exercise to achieve glucose levels that are near normal most of the time. As well as aiding in better control, self-monitoring has psychological advantages. One feels that one is in control of the disease rather than

controlled by it. Self-monitoring can soothe a child's anger and hostility over his condition. It is a positive action rather than just another shot to endure, another prick of the needle to bear. Sometimes if a child or his family are finding it exceptionally difficult to accept the diabetes, self-monitoring can be a significant help.

Q: *How?*
A: Refusal to accept the diabetes is masked very often by excessive, even morbid, preoccupation with the details of diabetes control. The anxiety and depression that result are related to how good the control is. Self-monitoring can make the control tighter and better. It also gives the child the idea that he is in the driver's seat.

Q: *Is special equipment needed?*
A: All that is required is a needle, lancet or automatic finger pricker, a drop of blood, a reagent strip (similar to those used for urine testing), and a watch with a second hand. A meter with which to read the strips is optional. Some can be read by eye. The procedure is very simple.

1. Wash hands in warm water. This removes any trace of sugar that could distort the reading. It also makes the skin warm and pink so that it is easy to squeeze out a drop of blood.
2. Choose a finger and milk it gently, forcing the blood into the tip.
3. Prick the side of the finger near the base of the nail lightly with an unused insulin needle, a lancet, or an automatic pricker. Do not prick the ball of the finger, which is very sensitive. (Do not allow anyone else to prick your child on the ball of the finger either, or it will discourage his own home blood monitoring.)
4. Squeeze out a drop of blood. (If there is any difficulty about getting a drop, do not poke and prod. Soak the finger in a cup of hand-hot water for a few minutes. The

blood will spurt easily after the slightest prick if the finger is warm.)

5. Turn the hand over so that the drop hangs down.
6. Allow it to drop neatly onto the end of the test strip.
7. Wait for exactly the length of time specified in the instructions. This is different for different ranges and for various brands of strips, so read the directions carefully before you begin.
8. Wipe or blot the strip with absorbent cotton or tissue, or wash with water, depending on the brand. There is some variation here as well, so read the directions carefully.
9. Compare the color with the chart, or read the results by placing the strip into the reflectance meter.
10. Record results in diary or notebook or put into memory bank of meter if your meter has one.

Q: *Is this procedure painful or unpleasant in any way?*
A: Many children find it preferable to urine testing. With a little practice, most manage to extract the blood drop painlessly. Without exception, they love using the meter and watching the number come up on the display screen. A child who is reluctant to test after realizing that it is not painful is probably apprehensive about the results.

It is important that your child not associate poor control with being "naughty." Test results should be discussed as "high," "normal," and "low" rather than as "good" and "bad." It is difficult to refrain from an approving word or smile when the test results are normal. After all, you are anxious about it and relieved when the test indicates that the blood glucose is not elevated. But every time you say "good boy" or "good girl" for a normal test, you reinforce the idea that poor results are his fault. Perhaps they are. Perhaps he has sneaked a candy bar, spent a sunny day in front of the television instead of out on his bike, or forgotten to take his evening shot until five minutes before dinner. Still, there will be many times when he has done everything right and the blood glucose will still be abnormal. There are many aspects of diabetes that are still not understood. No matter how he has behaved, it is better to encourage him to take an objective view of these tests, regarding them as a guide to diabetes management and not as a reflection on his behavior. Like the sailor who observes the weather in order to trim his sails, he is not fixing blame for the storm but using the information to steer a safe course.

Q: *Is it necessary to buy a meter to test blood at home?*
A: You can buy test strips that are read by eye alone. The end of the strip has a little pad that changes color according to the amount of glucose in the drop of blood. It is fairly easy to compare the color to the color chart on the bottle of strips. For a modest sum, you can purchase a color guide that helps to identify the colors with less chance of error.

If you use a meter, you insert the strip into it and press a button. The results appear in a display panel that tells you the blood glucose. More sophisticated meters retain a certain number of test results in their memory. They can average results as well, so that you can know at a glance how the diabetes is being controlled over a period of time. There is even a very small meter the shape and size of a fountain pen. You insert a test strip, put a drop of blood on the target area, and press a button. In 30 seconds, the results are displayed with no wiping, timing, or blotting. Make certain that you use the correct strip for your meter. Some available meters and their strips are:

Meter	*Strip*	*Manufacturer*
Accu-Check 11	Chemstrip	(Boehringer-Mannheim)
Betascan	Trendstrip	(Orange Medical)
Diascan	Diascan	(Home Diagnostics Inc)
Direct 30/30 Sensor	uses cartridges	(Elco)
ExacTech	ExacTech	(MediSense)
Glucometer 11	Glucostix	(Ames)
Glucoscan 3000	Glucoscan	(Lifescan)
One Touch	One Touch	(Lifescan)
Tracer 11	Tracer 11	(Boehringer-Mannheim)
Ultra	Ultra	(Home Diagnostics)

Q: *Is the meter more accurate than the strips you read by eye?*
A: A study made a few years ago indicates that they are equal in accuracy. In both cases, the skill of the user is the most important element. Some people prefer the meter because it is not open to interpretation or influenced by wishful thinking. However, cost is a factor for most people. Also, it is easy to get carried away by the glamour of the new technology and to forget that these gadgets are only as good as their users. Buying all the electronic gadgets in the world will not give your child normal blood glucose if he overeats, underexercises, or takes the wrong insulin dose.

Q: *My child is interested in computers. Are there computer programs about diabetes?*
A: Diabetes is a computer buff's dream. There are programs that require the child to put in his data, which is then analyzed and graphed and from which he can adjust his treatment. There are data management systems with which information can be put into your home computer and sent to your doctor's computer by telephone using a modem. These programs reinforce progress and give a psychological boost. If you can afford it, they add an element of fun, which is always beneficial.

Q: *Is it possible to buy diabetes equipment at a discount?*
A: Yes. Many mail-order pharmacies offer good discounts on diabetes equipment. Ask other people with diabetes in your area for the best place to shop. You may find that bulk buying saves you money. Before embarking on bulk buying of test strips, though, make certain that you will actually use that many before the expiration date.

Q: *How often should children do blood tests?*
A: This is a matter that you should discuss with your doctor. He will take into consideration the child's age, duration of diabetes, number of shots required, attitude of the patient, and many other factors. Naturally, the more tests one does, the more information one is building up regarding the blood glucose. However, it is not

only the number of tests that counts, but what you can do with the information received. If you have no one to guide you, and your child is on a one- or two-shot insulin regime, I suggest that you begin by testing once a day on weekdays and Saturdays with Sunday off for a treat.

Q: *What time of day is best?*
A: Vary the times. Let the child test before breakfast on Mondays, before dinner on Tuesdays, before bed on Wednesdays, after school (or midafternoon) on Thursdays, after dinner on Fridays, and before lunch on Saturdays. Or you could select two days a week and do four tests during those days at different times. One of these times could be at 2 or 3 o'clock in the morning, a time when blood glucose is lowest and nighttime reactions can occur. Record the results and bring them into your doctor's office for your next visit. He will be able to glean much useful information from them. Whatever testing program you decide to follow, try to keep a balanced view. Don't become a test-strip junkie, obsessed with diabetes. Your child's control may improve marginally from your zeal, but his attitude most certainly won't. Don't call him in from play to test. Don't embarrass him by insisting on a test before a meal in a restaurant or in someone else's house. In fact, never insist. Diabetes is his for life, and too much pressure when he is young could keep him from looking after himself when he is grown.

Q: *If he is willing to test regularly at home, why does he have to have a blood test in the lab as well? He dreads this test, especially when the blood is taken from his arm.*
A: The lab test takes several measurements that you cannot take at home. One important measurement is for glycosylated hemoglobin, or glycohemoglobin, usually abbreviated to GHb or HbA1c.

Q: *What is glycohemoglobin?*
A: Red blood cells carry the chemical hemoglobin. Normally,

only 6 percent of the hemoglobin has glucose molecules attached to it. The red blood cell has a life span of about three months. If the blood glucose has been running higher than usual over this period, a higher percentage of hemoglobin will have glucose attached. A satisfactory result is usually 6–9 percent. If this test is done every three months, you can see how valuable it is in determining the level of blood glucose over a long period.

Your child's fear of the blood test is probably rooted in his fear of being hurt when the blood is taken. Ask in the lab for an analgesic cream to be rubbed on the arm before the needle is inserted. This makes the arm less sensitive. It may be that you can buy such a cream in the drugstore for use before the lab test is scheduled. Also, some laboratories sell equipment for the taking of blood at home. You withdraw the sample and send it by mail. The results are returned by mail as well. Ask your doctor about the advisability of using such a service if your child continues to be frightened by having his blood taken.

Q: *Is it possible to be aware of changes in the blood glucose without testing?*
A: When blood glucose falls below normal, there are signs of an insulin reaction: confusion, sweating, irritability, pallor, trembling. When it rises quite a bit above normal, one feels tired, thirsty, often has a stomachache, and urinates frequently. If, however, the blood glucose is only slightly elevated, there are no obvious symptoms. This situation is dangerous and should be avoided.

Q: *Why is this state particularly dangerous?*
A: If the blood glucose is slightly elevated for long periods, the body adjusts. The child feels well, but the abnormal blood-glucose levels can give rise to complications in the future. Also, if he gets used to blood sugars that are consistently higher than normal, he may feel decidedly unwell and uneasy when returned to better control. This feeling may persist for some time. He may resist increasing his insulin because he does not want to "feel funny."

Q: *If a child tests his blood regularly, is there a need to do urine tests as well?*
A: Not on a daily basis. If he should become ill, however, it is important to know whether or not he is producing ketones. The blood tests will not show this. Only the urine tests will pick it up. Urine testing has rather fallen by the wayside since self-glucose monitoring was developed about ten years ago. Urine testing is a useful tool, though, especially in childhood, and should not be altogether abandoned in favor of the blood test.

Q: *Would you recommend the strips or the tablets for urine testing?*
A: If cost is not a factor, the strips are simpler and easier to keep. Tablets tend to crumble and discolor if they aren't kept absolutely dry and airtight. All reagents should be kept dry and the moisture-absorbent sachets in the bottles should not be discarded. But if you need to watch every penny and tablets are cheaper, don't worry. They are just as accurate. And after all, the point of the test is getting and using the information, not playing with the latest equipment.

Q: *Are all brands of strips equally accurate?*
A: All the brands that I have used appear to be equally accurate. If you plan to read them by eye, though, you must get the correct strip and not one meant to be read by machine. If your druggist does not have many customers with diabetes, he might not be aware of this, so be careful to read the literature before you buy anything. Also, different meters take different strips, so your strip must match your meter. If you purchase a meter, be sure to read all the literature that goes with it before buying new strips.

Q: *Is this equipment expensive?*
A: It is much less expensive than it was a few years ago. If cost is an important factor for you, buy the strips that are designed to be read by eye. You may find, though, that there are many special offers on meters or that your health-insurance policy will cover all

or part of the price. Remember that buying the latest and most sophisticated equipment will not control diabetes any better than the simplest. Most people enjoy the technology for its own sake: it takes the sting out of having to test every day, perhaps several times a day, if one has an interesting new gadget. But one of the best-controlled persons with diabetes I ever met was an elderly professor of medicine who, in his mid-seventies, had no trace of any diabetic complications. He had learned to control his diabetes thirty or forty years before, when none of these devices was available. He boiled his urine with Fehling's solution to test it for glucose, but that was the only scientific measurement he could make then. Still, his diligence in performing this test, his diet, and his refusal to let his diabetes keep him from pursuing his career or keep him from traveling, which he loved, was an example of what one could do with knowledge and determination. The technology available to diabetics now is enormous, but the most important aspects of control are still knowledge and determination.

Q: *Is the cost of blood-testing strips justified?*
A: Absolutely. It enables one to make small changes in routine, increase or decrease the insulin, adjust the diet, or step up the exercise according to the amount of glucose in the bloodstream. If one were to depend on urine testing alone, it would be necessary to consider the fact that the glucose levels observed may not be a true indication of the actual level in the body. The urine you have tested may have been in the bladder for several hours. If urine tests are the only guide to insulin adjustment, they are a much rougher guide. They do not help to fine-tune control to keep levels below 180 mg/dl.

Q: *What do you do if you find that there is a high glucose reading before breakfast?*
A: If the child is on routine insulin therapy, taking a combination of Regular and NPH or lente insulins twice a day, increase the NPH/lente in the *evening* dose. This covers the nighttime. Test again the next morning. If it is lower, you have done the right

thing. However, if it is higher, and especially if the child complains of a headache, another explanation must be considered. If the evening dose of insulin was too *high* rather than too low, the blood glucose may have gone too low during the night. This would have gone unnoticed during sleep. To protect itself from hypoglycemia, the body would have released into the bloodstream extra glucose from the liver. The blood test in the morning reflects this. This is a common phenomenon called "rebound hyperglycemia." The headache is your clue that a mild reaction took place during the night. In this case, you should reduce the dose of NPH/lente that evening.

Q: *Suppose the reading the next morning is lower but still not normal. What do you do then?*
A: If you increased the dose to improve glucose levels and it worked, just increase the dose a little more. If, on the other hand, a decrease brought about better control, then decrease the insulin again.

Q: *By how many units should you change the dose?*
A: Ask your doctor or diabetes educator. There is a great variation in response. If you cannot get advice, move cautiously, changing the insulin one unit at a time until you get a satisfactory level in the morning. The morning glucose is generally the most difficult to control. There is a natural rise of blood glucose toward dawn that is difficult to estimate. Also, it is hard to know whether a high blood glucose in the morning is due to too much or too little insulin unless you are willing to test the blood at 2 or 3 A.M. If this problem persists, this is the only way to sort it out. With a young child, it is often possible to do a finger prick without awakening him. If this test shows levels below normal, it is likely that reducing the evening dose will bring about improvement in the morning.

If it proves impossible to get normal readings in the morning on two shots a day, your doctor may consider adding a third shot at bedtime. If this happens, it is not a reflection on your care or a sign that the diabetes is getting worse. It is just easier to control rebound hyperglycemia by giving the medium-acting insulin at bedtime instead of before dinner.

Q: *Suppose that the child is taking one shot a day in the morning, and it isn't possible to change the evening dose. What do you do then?*
A: Increase the Regular insulin in the morning to lower the blood glucose at once. However, if you find that he is having a reaction midmorning, you could try increasing the circulation instead of increasing the dose. Rub the injection site for five minutes or warm it gently. This will help the insulin to circulate more quickly and bring down the blood glucose without causing hypoglycemia a few hours later. If you find that the morning levels are consistently high, consult your doctor. He may recommend a change to a two-injection routine in order to improve control.

Q: *What do you do if the morning glucose reading is below normal?*
A: Solve the immediate problem by giving the child a sweet drink like orange juice to bring the glucose levels up to normal. Then lower the evening dose of NPH/lente.

Q: *Do you give the orange juice before the shot?*
A: Yes. The idea is to raise the glucose levels before the next dose of insulin takes effect.

Q: *What do you do if this problem persists?*
A: Consult your doctor. He may want to review the dosage and perhaps make some changes.

Q: *How do you treat a high glucose reading before lunch?*
A: Increase the morning dose of Regular insulin the next morning.

Q: *What about a low reading before lunch?*
A: Give sugar right away followed by a snack. The next morning, reduce the morning dose of Regular insulin.

Q: *What do you do if there is a high reading before the evening meal?*
A: When you give the evening shot, increase the circulation by massage or gentle heat. If the child is willing, send him out for some vigorous exercise before dinner. Sometimes just a run around the block or ten minutes on his bike will bring it down. Then increase the NPH/lente the next morning.

Q: *What do you do if there is a reaction before dinner?*
A: Give sugar. Decrease the NPH/lente the next morning to avoid a repetition. If this persists, it may be necessary to move the meal to an earlier time.

Q: *How do you treat a high reading before bedtime?*
A: Increase the evening dose of Regular insulin the next day.

Q: *What do you do if the child has a reaction before going to bed?*
A: Give sugar. Reduce the evening dose of Regular insulin the next evening.

Q: *I know some parents who were warned in the hospital never to change their child's insulin dose. What do you advise in that situation?*
A: That is very difficult to say. It is not possible to get good diabetic control if you cannot vary the insulin dose to keep the blood glucose normal. There is not much sense in testing the child's blood or urine for glucose if there is nothing that you can do about it. I think that the best thing to do in that case is to see the doctor again and ask him why he has prohibited changing the dose. Perhaps if he can see that the parents have a fair understanding of diabetes control, he might feel more confident about

allowing changes. I was once at a conference for parents of children with diabetes when this question came up. A woman asked it of the distinguished British pediatrician who was addressing the meeting, a man with many years of experience as the head of a large and famous specialist clinic and the author of several books on diabetes. His reply was short, and I remember it well: "If your consultant [specialist] will not allow you to change your child's insulin, change your consultant."

Q: *Is there any other way of controlling the diabetes other than increasing or decreasing the insulin?*
A: One simple trick is to use time to your advantage. If the reading is slightly too high, give the shot an hour before the meal instead of half an hour before. That way, the insulin action will be stronger before more food is consumed.

Q: *Normally, what should the time lag be between the injection and the meal?*
A: Aim for thirty minutes. Sometimes it is difficult to do this in the morning when everyone seems to be rushing out to school or work, but it will give better control. It is worthwhile to get up a little earlier and do the test and injection before dressing.

Q: *I understand that a reading between 72 mg/dl and 126 mg/dl is normal, but at what point shall I begin manipulating the insulin? If it is 145 or 160, shall I add a unit?*
A: Unless otherwise instructed by the doctor or unless you are on a multiple-injection regime using a pen, button, or pump, I wouldn't add any insulin unless the blood glucose is 180 mg/dl. With readings between 126 and 179, give the shot earlier, try to increase circulation or absorption, or, if the child is reasonably plump, reduce the carbohydrates in the meal by 10 grams.

Q: *What if it is lower than 72 mg/dl?*
A: Low blood glucose is easier to deal with in some ways because there is no time to worry about what to do. If a reaction

threatens, you must act immediately by giving sugar. You should do this if the reading is lower than 70 mg/dl or if the child feels the symptoms of an insulin reaction.

Q: *What is the reason for insulin reactions?*
A: A reaction can occur if the insulin is not balanced by the carbohydrate intake. If, for example, the child has his usual shot of insulin in the morning but then plays a vigorous game without taking any extra carbohydrates, his blood glucose may drop too low. If a meal or snack is forgotten, there may be too much insulin in the bloodstream and too little food for it to work on. Balance and regularity are the keys to diabetes control.

Q: *Why regularity?*
A: Diabetes control is easier if the child gets up at the same time every day, has his meals at the same time, and goes to bed at the same time every evening. Nothing will throw the diabetes off balance more quickly than missed snacks, late meals, or staying in bed very late on weekend and holiday mornings.

Q: *If my child has a bad reaction in the night, should I keep him home from school the next day?*
A: You will have to judge the state of his health in the morning. It is likely that he will not remember the events of the previous night even though the rest of the family are still upset. He may have a headache. His blood glucose will undoubtedly be high. This is only temporary. It will drop later in the day. If he wants to go to school, I would be inclined to let him, but I would give him extra carbohydrates to take if should he feel low again. (This is unlikely but it will make you feel better.) You should telephone the school and ask them to let you know if he becomes unwell. (This probably won't happen either, but it will make you feel better.) Insulin reactions are usually much more distressing to the parent than to the child.

Q: *What can I do to ensure that it will not recur?*
A: Review the events of the previous days in your mind. Were there small signals that you overlooked? Did he have several

episodes of mild hypoglycemia that you counteracted by giving an extra snack or moving up his mealtime? Did he eat all his bedtime snack on the evening of the reaction? Was it large enough? Did he use up more energy than usual in play that day? Could his insulin be reduced without sending up his blood glucose? If you think it could, try it. If you have chosen your physician wisely, you should be able to call on him for advice at this stage. Remember that self-monitoring of glucose is a faithful guide if done accurately. It is these test results that enable you to make an informed, intelligent decision. It is necessary to keep in mind, however, that the diabetes will become unstable at times even though you have been doing all the right things. Sometimes the insulin is absorbed more quickly than usual. There is no way of knowing this in advance. Frequent severe reactions, however, are uncommon in a child whose diabetes is well controlled.

Q: *Are seizures common during a reaction?*
A: Some children have a seizure if the blood glucose drops suddenly. Of course, some children have a seizure if their temperature rises very high. Others never do. A seizure is very upsetting to the parent, but there is no evidence that it does permanent damage to the child. If your child has a seizure, you should inform your doctor at once and reduce the child's insulin.

Q: *Are reactions more common at night?*
A: It is possible that they are because the blood glucose is at its lowest ebb during the early hours of the morning. But it is more likely that it just seems that way because no one is awake to recognize the warning signs and take prompt action. Also, everything seems worse in the middle of the night. Parents are not at their best, awakened from sleep, trying to cope with an unreasonable child without any warning.

Q: *How long does it take after sugar is given for the reaction to abate?*
A: In a mild reaction where warning signs are noted and sugar

eaten, the symptoms will go away in a short time. A headache may linger, though.

Q: *How do you cope with a baby or very young child who cannot recognize the symptoms?*
A: The parent must be extremely observant and vigilant about sticking to the diabetic regime. Keeping to exact mealtimes and snack times will help to keep a balance between insulin and food. Keep a watchful eye on the child if he should suddenly stop playing and become quiet. Many young children become pale if their glucose levels fall. Err on the side of caution. If you think that he might be starting to react, give him a sweet drink immediately. If he recovers himself in a few minutes, you will know that you were right. If he continues to act strangely, keep him under observation. With small bodies, things happen quickly. Perhaps he is coming down with an infection. If you are uncertain, test his blood. You will find a blood test a great source of comfort in times of uncertainty.

Q: *I think that my child's blood glucose is higher on days when we go to the doctor than on other days. Is this a coincidence?*
A: It is difficult to measure stress, but it is common knowledge that stress affects the blood glucose. I don't think that this is a coincidence. This is another reason for testing regularly at home. If a single test done at the lab on the day of the visit to the doctor were the only guide to insulin dosage, most persons with diabetes would be taking too much insulin.

Q: *Can school pressures upset the diabetes control?*
A: Any stress can raise the blood glucose. This is part of the body's mechanism for fighting back. However, your child should not be encouraged to use his diabetes as an excuse for poor school performance. Missing school days certainly has an effect on grades. You can play a significant role in ensuring that the usual illnesses of childhood do not upset the diabetes control and cause him to miss extra days of school.

Q: *Can a minor illness like a cold upset the diabetes?*
A: Generally, at the first sign of an illness, even a minor one, blood glucose goes up. Sometimes, even with a minor infection, the blood glucose rises quite high and ketones may be formed.

Q: *Why does this happen?*
A: Insulin is a storage hormone. If the body lacks insulin, it cannot store glucose, protein, or fat. When fat molecules are broken down (because they cannot be stored), they release fatty acids, or ketones, into the bloodstream. If the body is overwhelmed with ketones, serious illness, even death, can result. When your child first developed diabetes, he was probably producing large amounts of ketones. He was thirsty all the time, urinating copiously, perhaps tired and lethargic. Other signs of ketone production are abdominal pain, vomiting, deep, sighing breathing, and eventually coma. The presence of ketones indicates that insulin is required urgently.

Q: *How do you know when ketones are present?*
A: They are detectable in the urine. At the first sign of illness, test the urine for ketones. Even if the test is negative, continue to test the urine several times a day until the illness has passed. Sometimes, in their enthusiasm for blood testing, people forget that urine testing still has a part to play in diabetes control, especially during illness.

Q: *What should be done if ketones are present?*
A: Give more insulin.

Q: *How much more?*
A: Call your doctor if possible. If you cannot get medical advice, increase by 2 units of Regular insulin and test often to see whether this is enough. If the child is feverish, you will probably need to give more Regular insulin. During illness, it is a good idea to give extra shots even if the usual regime is one or two shots a day. One or two extra shots are generally required to cope with the in-

creased glucose levels produced by a feverish illness. A combination of blood and urine tests should be your guide if you cannot get medical help.

Q: *What happens if the child can barely eat enough food to cope with his normal insulin dose and won't eat anything extra to cope with the extra insulin?*
A: Give him light foods that are tolerated easily when ill: gelatin desserts, fruit and fruit juice, regular soda, lemonade, tea with sugar, Gatorade, applesauce, ice cream, etc. These foods are high in easily assimilated sugars. Give fluids often. A sick child should drink at least a half-cup of fluid every hour.

Q: *What can be done if he cannot take enough exchanges for a meal?*
A: Don't worry about making up enough for a meal. Offer food often. Let him eat or drink one exchange an hour if that is all he can tolerate.

Q: *What should I do if he refuses all foods or vomits?*
A: If he will not eat or drink, consider it an emergency. You need medical help. If you cannot get any advice, take him to the emergency room of the nearest hospital, especially if he is vomiting. Do not delay. A child with diabetes who is manufacturing ketones and who is vomiting needs professional medical treatment.

Q: *Shall I stop the insulin if he is vomiting and cannot keep down the food at all?*
A: No. *Never stop the insulin.* An insulin-dependent person with diabetes needs insulin every day. More insulin, not less, is needed during illness. Urine tests will bear this out as well. If he is vomiting, he will be showing both glucose and ketones. Therefore, he needs more insulin. The urine tests are your best guide during illness. Even if you are blood-testing regularly, using a pump, and in possession of the latest electronic meter that averages the test results at the flick of a button, you still must return to urine testing for ketones during illness.

Q: *Is it likely that my child will be hospitalized more often now that he has diabetes?*
A: No, not at all. By observing a few simple rules, the child with diabetes can be looked after at home in the same way as other members of the family. The important points to remember are:

1. Act quickly. Do not wait to see how things develop. Things develop rapidly with children, and all problems are more easily solved in the early stages.
2. More, not less, insulin is required during illness, no matter how little food is eaten.
3. Test the urine for glucose and ketones several times a day.
4. Test the blood glucose several times a day.
5. Switch to a light diet, even though sugary foods are usually avoided.
6. Give plenty of fluids.

Q: *Now that my child has diabetes, will he become ill more often?*
A: There is no evidence to show that he will be ill more often. When my child was first diagnosed, the doctors gave me so many instructions about what to do during illness that I had the impression that she would be down with everything that came along. On the contrary, she is almost never ill and has had milder bouts of the usual childhood diseases than my other children. What does happen, though, is that any illness, especially a virus infection with a fever, upsets the diabetes control and more insulin and careful monitoring are required. Should the illness require the attention of a specialist, he or she must always consult the diabetes physician before any treatment.

Q: *What happens if my child has to be hospitalized with, for example, a tonsillectomy? Is this a problem?*
A: It can be. If your pediatrician recommends a tonsillectomy, I would consider it very carefully, discuss it thoroughly with him, and if possible get a second opinion. In most children, tonsils

shrink after the age of seven and give much less trouble. This is one operation that is subject to fashion. A generation ago, they were done routinely on every child with repeated throat and middle-ear infections, but the incidence of them now is much less. However, if you are convinced that the operation is necessary, the doctor in charge should consult with the physician in charge of the diabetes treatment so that adequate arrangements can be made for your child's care while in the hospital.

Q: *Is there anything that parents can do?*
A: Parents can and should do a great deal. Make sure that your child's blood sugars are as near normal as you can get them before the operation. This will promote healing. Bring all your equipment with you. You can't expect the hospital to have special injectors or any other equipment that he is used to. See the dietician and agree on a meal plan for your child. Most important, *stay with the child.* Insist on this. Be tactful, but be firm. Ask the doctor to instruct the nurses involved that the child's glucose tests and his insulin are to be administered by you. Check everything, especially the contents of syringes. Don't assume that the ward nurses know anything about diabetes. They don't. It is not that they are stupid or poorly trained; it is just that insulin-dependent diabetes is a highly specialized subject. A common problem in hospitals is that meals and insulin injections are not properly synchronized. You cannot sit idly by and allow a nurse to inject your child with insulin at 3 P.M. when you know that supper isn't served until 5 P.M.

Q: *What happens if the child is rushed into the hospital for an emergency such as an accident and there is no time to prepare?*
A: You have to think on your feet. If your child has had an accident, he might be in shock. This will certainly upset the diabetes control. Get in touch with your diabetes physician urgently. His presence is required at the hospital. Don't allow the child to be starved in preparation for surgery unless you are confident that the staff understand how to deal with an insulin-dependent person with diabetes. He will probably have to be hooked up to an IV for

both insulin and glucose in order to stabilize his blood sugar. Try not to make a nuisance of yourself and alienate the doctors and nurses, but do not leave your child's bedside until you are certain that the medical staff are taking his diabetes into consideration.

If a major accident occurs with serious wounds, discuss with the doctor the advisability of contacting the Curatec Wound Care Center at the University of Minnesota. The Center specializes in the healing of wounds under difficult conditions. The number to call is 1-612-625-5919.

Q: *My child seems to complain a lot about stomachaches now that he has diabetes. Is this common?*

A: Stomachaches can be symptomatic of a number of conditions: low blood sugar, high blood sugar, lactose intolerance (inability to digest milk sugar), excessive sorbitol, and others. Test his glucose levels more frequently and tell the doctor about his complaints. If it is lactose intolerance, a milk-free diet will help. If he cannot take much sorbitol, you will have to cut down on the amount of sugar-free candy that he eats. (This is a good idea anyway. These products should be used sparingly.)

Q: *Will the diabetes affect other aspects of health care like dental hygiene?*

A: Diabetes does affect the teeth, and a person who has diabetes needs to take particular care of teeth and gums. Since abnormal glucose levels affect the blood vessels throughout the body, the tiny blood vessels in the gums can also be affected. If the gums become diseased because of faulty circulation in these small vessels, the roots of the teeth and the bone in which they are held are affected. Improper care can lead to the gum disease called gingivitis and result in early loss of teeth. All children should attend the dentist regularly, but for the child with diabetes, it is vital. However, try to keep your child's schedule in mind when arranging for dental work to be done. Make sure that it does not interfere with his lunch or snack time. If a dental appointment is scheduled just before lunch and the child has to wait a long time for his turn, his blood glucose might drop below normal. If he has to wait for a long time after treatment before he can eat, it could cause a problem. Tell the dentist that he has diabetes and must have his meals on time. Also, if he has to have a tooth extracted or any work done under a general anesthetic, this must be done in a hospital. The dentist should confer with the doctor who is looking after the diabetes before any such dental work is undertaken.

Q: *Can the child with diabetes have a local anesthetic for dental treatment?*
A: He can have an injection of novocaine, vidocaine, etc. For any other anesthetic (gas, for example) the dentist should confer with the physician in charge.

Q: *Can the child with diabetes take ordinary medicines? I am thinking of the sugary solutions in which children's antibiotics are mixed, and also of cough syrups.*
A: The most urgent requirement of the sick child is to get well. If there is an alternative to sugary medicines, your doctor can prescribe them. There are sugar-free cough and cold mixtures on the market, but there may not be sugar-free substitutes for other medications. In any case, it is more important to clear the infection than to count the carbohydrates. A teaspoon of a child's antibiotic contains only 5 grams of sugar anyway. If the child needs an antibiotic, it is likely that he has a fever, that his blood glucose is elevated, and that he is producing ketones as well. He will therefore be taking extra insulin that day, which will cover the sugar in the medicine.

Q: *I have heard that girls get an itchy discharge from the vagina when they have diabetes. Is this common and what causes it?*
A: The condition is not uncommon when the diabetes is first discovered. It is caused by organisms that thrive in a sugary environment. It is not serious and will generally clear up when the blood glucose is lowered. If it is bothersome, the doctor can pre-

scribe a cream. If the condition recurs after insulin therapy has been established, it is a sign that the blood glucose is still too high. More frequent finger pricks are needed as a guide to adjusting the insulin to keep the glucose levels near normal.

Q: *Can boys get a similar infection?*
A: They can, but it is less common. The end of the penis can become sore and the foreskin thickened. This, too, is caused by high concentrations of sugar. Keeping the diabetes under control will ensure that the urine stays free from sugar and the genital area free from these infections.

Q: *My child complains sometimes of blurred vision. What is the cause of this?*
A: Changes in the levels of blood glucose, either rising or falling, can cause blurred vision. This is not a serious condition. It is usually temporary, but it should be reported to your doctor. Check the glucose levels often with finger pricks and try to bring the diabetes under steadier control.

Q: *I know that diabetes can cause blindness. Does this happen to children?*
A: Diabetes is the largest cause of blindness in young and older adults, and diabetic retinopathy is one of the serious complications of long-term diabetes. Still, less than 10 percent of people with diabetes become blind, and in the last few years, there has been marked success in treating the retinopathy with laser surgery before loss of vision. In order for this treatment to be successful, though, the retinopathy must be diagnosed at an early stage. If it is left too long, there is no way to prevent blindness. It is extremely important, therefore, to have a regular eye examination by a qualified ophthalmologist (not an optometrist) in order to keep a close watch on the small blood vessels of the retina and effects on the vitreous fluid of the eye. Premature cataracts may also develop, affecting vision. This is an area where one should never take a chance. Make certain that your child's appointments with the ophthalmologist are kept scrupulously.

Q: *What about the child who wears glasses?*
A: The optometrist who measures your child's vision for glasses should be told that the child has become diabetic. Optometrists can sometimes pick up early signs of retinopathy and will advise you to see your ophthalmologist. However, just because the optometrist examines your child's eyes and reports no abnormalities does not mean that you needn't check further. The ophthalmologist has more sensitive equipment at his command, such as dye photographs of the retina, which can detect abnormalities at an earlier stage.

Q: *Is laser surgery expensive or difficult?*
A: The expense will depend on local conditions and on your insurance coverage. It is a procedure that has become more common in the last few years. It is not really a surgical operation. The patient looks into a machine at what appears to be a very bright light but what is actually a laser beam that seals the damaged blood vessels so that they stop leaking. There is no pain involved, but the procedure is frightening to many people. The best medicine in this case is, of course, preventive. Eye problems are more likely after long periods of poor diabetes control.

Q: *What about kidney complications?*
A: Thirty to 40 percent of all people with kidney damage in the United States have diabetes. This does not mean, of course, that your child will suffer from kidney disease. There has been much research into diabetic kidney disease in the last few years, and the results are encouraging. Every time your child attends the diabetes specialist, he will have his urine tested for traces of protein, which would indicate that the kidneys are not functioning efficiently. If protein is detected, a special diet or tighter glucose control may be recommended. Certain drugs used to control high blood pressure may be prescribed. Recent research indicates that this treatment inhibits kidney disease. The medical scientists are very hopeful that, in the future, fewer people with diabetes will develop these complications. Meanwhile, we are all advised to

drink more water. Eight glasses a day is recommended by nutritionists. This is a good habit for everyone, and especially for the person with diabetes. Be careful, too, not to serve your child excessive amounts of protein. We Americans tend to eat more protein than we need, and there is some evidence to show that the kidneys have to work harder when a large amount of protein is consumed. Discuss this with your dietician or nutritionist. A three-ounce serving of meat or poultry probably provides enough protein for a meal. Carbohydrate snacks such as popcorn or waffles should be eaten more often than peanut butter or cheese, which are protein foods. Milk intake should never exceed one quart a day.

Q: *What about nerve damage? Isn't this a possible complication?*
A: It is possible for nerve damage or neuropathy to develop. That is one reason why people with diabetes are advised not to go barefoot and to wear well-fitting shoes. Neuropathy reduces sensitivity, and small injuries to the feet may go unnoticed. It is difficult to prevent a young child from running about barefoot in the house or on the beach, but certainly parents can ensure that footwear is of good quality and properly fitted. Soft leather is the best. No one ever suffered damage to his health by wearing ugly, cheap, or unfashionable clothes or big brother's hand-me-downs, but shoes are something else. Avoid foot problems such as corns and calluses, cuts, and bruises. These are less likely to heal quickly if the blood glucose is elevated. Also, the foot is less sensitive to heat and cold if the blood supply is reduced or if the nerves are damaged. Ice skates and ski boots should be of good quality and fit well to allow adequate circulation. Socks should be of natural fibers, cotton or wool, and be free of seams. Don't darn them if they develop holes. Replace them. The stitching can cause irritation.

There has been a promising line of research in diabetic neuropathy in the last few years. It has been discovered that the enzyme aldose reductase, which is activated by the diabetic body in order to get rid of excess glucose, creates a process whereby the sugar alcohol sorbitol is trapped in the cells, where it damages the nerves. If the aldose reductase enzyme could be inhibited, the levels of sorbitol would decrease. This is a most exciting line of study, and one that may have important developments for the future, possibly affecting other complications of diabetes as well.

Q: *I have heard that some people with diabetes have had to have limbs amputated. Does this still happen?*
A: It happens less and less as we know more about diabetes and how to control it.

Q: *What causes these complications?*
A: There is evidence to suggest that they are the consequences of long-term abnormalities in blood-glucose levels. There is also some evidence to show that people who are well controlled from the onset of the disease will be less likely to develop these complications. That is why it is very important that you teach your child responsible attitudes toward his diabetes. He should regard the specialist clinic as a helpful place, the diagnostic tests as preventive rather than unpleasant, and the adjustment of his insulin to keep normal glucose levels as part of life.

The National Institutes of Health has a long-term study under way to determine the effects of tight glucose control on the complications of diabetes. It is called the Diabetes Control and Complications Trial, or DCCT. The first results will be published in 1991. The NIH has hundreds of volunteers with diabetes all over the country who are being monitored to provide data for this exhaustive study, the largest such project ever undertaken. There may be certain advantages in volunteering if more are required. All volunteers are given free equipment for the duration of the study, which is several years. Some will have the opportunity to try multiple injection therapy or a pump. All will be looked after by specialists who are extremely interested in diabetes, and it is an opportunity to learn more about the disease and to improve control at the same time that one is contributing to the sum total of medical knowledge.

If you are interested in learning more about this project, you can call 1-800-522-DCCT toll-free. The number in Canada is 1-800-533-DCCT. To become a volunteer, your child has to be over thirteen, have had insulin-dependent diabetes for less than five years, and be taking no more than one or two shots a day. When you dial the DCCT number, you'll hear a prerecorded message asking you to reply to certain questions. If your answers indicate that you meet their requirements, they will write to you with further details.

4
Food Plan

Q: *Why does my child have to be on a special diet?*
A: Insulin production is automatic in the healthy body. Every time one eats, the correct amount of insulin is released. When this process breaks down, the person develops diabetes and insulin must be injected at least once a day. As the amount of insulin each time is fairly constant, so the amount of carbohydrates eaten should be approximately the same every day.

Q: *What exactly are carbohydrates?*
A: Food is designated as carbohydrates, protein, and fat.

Carbohydrates consist of sugars and starches. Examples of carbohydrate foods are cereals, bread, cake, cookies, crackers, rice, pasta (spaghetti, macaroni, noodles, etc.), barley, pulses like lentils, peas and beans, potatoes, fruit, and milk products. Carbohydrate foods represent the bulk of our diet. They are generally the most filling and also the cheapest part of the food we eat.

Q: *I thought that it is sugar that needs insulin. Bread and milk aren't sweet. Why do they need insulin?*
A: All carbohydrates are broken down into simple sugars by the

digestive system, beginning with the saliva in the mouth and continuing into the stomach and the large and small intestines. The main simple sugar carried in the blood is glucose, and insulin is required for its use.

Q: *If this is so, then why can't the person with diabetes avoid carbohydrates and eat only protein and fat to avoid the need for insulin?*
A: Besides the fact that insulin has uses other than the metabolism of sugars, carbohydrate foods are necessary for good health and growth. A person who attempted to live on proteins and fats alone would not be well nourished. He would always be hungry and his kidneys would be overworked. Bread, fruit, and dairy products are an important part of our diet. The diet of the child with diabetes is no different from that of any other child except that the complex carbohydrates should be used rather than simple sugars.

Q: *What are complex carbohydrates?*
A: Complex carbohydrates are the starchy foods. They take longer to break down into simple sugars. The body has to work harder to digest them (break them down).

Q: *What proportion of the diet should be carbohydrate?*
A: Total calories should comprise 50 to 60 percent carbohydrates, 25 to 30 percent fat, and 15 to 20 percent protein.

Q: *Is a vegetarian diet suitable for persons with diabetes?*
A: Yes.

Q: *Is it suitable for children?*
A: It can be if sufficient protein is eaten. If your child is a vegetarian, the dietician in your specialist clinic can help you to devise a suitable vegetarian food plan.

Q: *What sort of diet is suitable?*
A: Let's stop talking about "diet," which has a negative connotation. Instead, let's call it a "food plan." A food plan for people with diabetes is really a good food plan for everyone in the family. In fact, this is really the secret of success in this aspect of diabetes control. Instead of restricting the child to a food plan that is suitable for him, change the eating habits of the entire family to conform to those recommended for him. You will find that everyone will benefit.

Q: *In what way?*
A: There may be less obesity and risk of heart disease. Possibly, there will be fewer bowel disorders.

Q: *But doesn't my child with diabetes have to be on a special diet?*
A: He needs to be on a food plan that measures the amount of carbohydrates, fat, and protein eaten, not necessarily one that restricts it unduly. Special diabetic diets that severely restricted the amount of carbohydrate and increased the amount of fat are no longer used. Modern diabetic food plans are suitable for everyone. After many years of studying the relationship between illness and nutrition, scientists have recommended that everyone reduce sugar, fat, and salt and increase fiber. This applies to all of us.

Q: *How does this type of eating compare with our present diet?*
A: Let's consider sugar. The average person in the United States consumes 5 ounces of sugar a day, about 10 tablespoons. Some of this is used for sweetening coffee and tea, but most of it is hidden in the processed foods we buy.

Q: *Do you mean cakes and desserts?*
A: Yes, but also in breakfast cereals, canned vegetables and meats, bouillon cubes, soft drinks, cookies, bread, sauces, soups,

gravy mixes, etc. Almost every food made in a factory contains sugar, even though it does not taste sweet.

Q: *Why is sugar put into foods that aren't meant to be sweet?*
A: It is used as a preservative and to improve flavor.

Q: *So giving up sugar in coffee and tea isn't sufficient to reduce sugar intake, is it?*
A: It will help, but it will not reduce it sufficiently unless we reduce the amount of processed food we consume as well, or at least choose those manufactured foods that are low in sugar.

Q: *What about fat? Why should fat reduction be important for people with diabetes?*
A: For the same reason that it is important for everyone: because there is strong evidence that reduction in fat will bring about reduced levels of heart disease. Since persons with diabetes are already at increased risk of heart disease, it seems sensible to reduce fat intake even in children.

Q: *What about salt?*
A: Salt reduction is usually recommended where there is a risk of high blood pressure. Since diabetes can cause narrowing of the blood vessels, which leads to high blood pressure (hypertension) in adult life, and since there is a link between high blood pressure and disease, it is reasonable to reduce salt as well.

Q: *I have heard a lot about fiber in the last few years. What exactly is fiber, and how does it fit into a diabetic food plan?*
A: Fiber is that part of plant food that cannot be digested. It passes through the body and is eliminated. If it is removed from the food by modern refining methods, the food is assimilated more quickly and with less effort. The body doesn't have to work as hard. Muscles designed to deal with fibrous food become lax,

and often problems ensue such as chronic constipation, gallbladder trouble, and bowel disease.

Q: *Are people with diabetes more likely to suffer from these diseases?*
A: Not necessarily, but these dietary changes are recommended for everyone. Now that you have a child with diabetes in your family, you are at a crossroads in your life where changes in diet are required. This is a good time to introduce healthier eating habits to your family that might have a salutary effect on their future.

Also, as regards the child with diabetes, fiber-rich foods take longer to be digested than those from which the fiber has been removed, so they are distinctly better at controlling the blood glucose. Glucose levels rise more steeply after eating easily digested carbohydrates, simple sugars like those in candy, soda, and sweet desserts, than they do after eating whole-grain bread and oatmeal that the body has to work harder to digest. You can use this natural fact of metabolism to help keep glucose levels more even.

Q: *What, then, is a good food plan for my child?*
A: When a child is first diagnosed as having diabetes, it is usual for him to be admitted to the hospital for stabilization. Often, his diabetes has caused him to lose weight, even become dehydrated, and he is in need of specialized care for a few days. Insulin therapy will be started and the child and his parents will have several consultations with the doctor, the diabetes educator, and the dietician. The dietician will discuss the family's eating patterns and generally recommend changes. Then the child will be given a food plan designed especially for him. This food plan will take into consideration his age, weight, preferences and dislikes, family circumstances, ethnic background, and lifestyle. It will be worked out in conjunction with the amounts and times of his insulin shots. The carbohydrates, fat, and protein required will be measured and the amounts worked out for every meal.

Q: *Is this very complicated?*
A: Not at all. The dietician will show you how many grams of carbohydrates, fat, and protein are required for each meal and will help you to work out which foods are the most suitable. She will also show you how to count exchanges.

Q: *What are exchanges?*
A: An exchange is a measured portion of food. The exchange system divides foods into groups. Foods within one group can be exchanged for others in the same group. It is an easy way of adding up the food values. If you didn't think of portions as exchangeable, you would spend more time in the kitchen weighing and measuring. As you work with the exchange system, you will become experienced at judging quantities at a glance. Eating in restaurants or in someone's home will become less of a problem, and you will become more able to help your child to resume his normal activities.

Q: *How does the exchange system work?*
A: There are six food groups: milk; vegetables; fruit; bread, rice, and starchy vegetables; meat; and fat.

(Since everyone, even young children, is being advised to reduce saturated fat, the following exchange lists contain milk values for skim milk. If your doctor wants your child to have full-cream milk, you should add 2 fat exchanges for every cup.)

Milk and Milk Products

One exchange of skim milk (1 cup) contains 12 grams of carbohydrates, 8 grams of protein, and a trace of fat. It has 80 calories. The following amounts of milk products equal 1 exchange. This means that they can be exchanged for 1 cup of milk because they have approximately the same food value:

powdered dry milk (nonfat) .... 1 cup
canned, evaporated skim milk .... ½ cup

buttermilk .... 1 cup
unflavored low-fat yogurt (made from skim milk) . 1 cup

Vegetables

Green and yellow vegetables are leading sources of many vitamins and minerals. They also contain fiber. If they are not overcooked, their vivid colors are attractive to children. Serve as many vegetables raw as is suitable. Young children usually love raw carrots, celery, cucumber, peppers, and tomatoes. Mine have always liked vegetables of all sorts, preferring to eat even cabbage, brussels sprouts, broccoli, and asparagus raw or lightly steamed. Even spinach can be eaten raw if desired. Spinach leaves torn up with lettuce make a salad look more interesting and have a delicious flavor. Raw beets and brussels sprouts are delicious grated and served in little mounds on a salad plate with dressing. The following is a list of vegetables for 1 exchange. The quantity is ½ cup. This amount contains approximately 5 grams of carbohydrates, 2 grams of protein, and 28 calories. Remember that the salad dressing or any butter or margarine served with vegetables is not a vegetable exchange. These items are fats.

Artichokes
Asparagus
Bamboo shoots
Beets
Broccoli
Brussels sprouts
Cabbage
Carrots
Cauliflower
Celery
Chicory
Chives
Cucumbers
Endive
Eggplant
Escarole
Greens (beet greens, chards, collards, dandelion greens, kale, mustard greens, spinach, turnip greens)
Jicama
Lettuce
Mushrooms
Okra
Onions
Parsley

Peppers (green, red, or yellow)
Radishes
Rutabaga
Sauerkraut
String beans, green beans, or yellow beans
Summer squash (crookneck or other varieties)
Tomatoes
Tomato juice
Vegetable juice
Watercress

Fruit

Fruits are good sources of vitamins, minerals, and fiber too, as well as being the favorite foods of most children. Please note that while vegetable juices were counted as 1 exchange the same as ½ cup of vegetables, fruit juices are not. Fruit juices contain sugar that is quickly absorbed into the bloodstream. They should be used when a rapid increase in the blood glucose is desired (for example, when the glucose level is too low) but not too often at other times. One fruit exchange contains 10 grams of carbohydrates and approximately 40 calories.

Apple	1 small
Applesauce	½ cup
Apricots	2 medium
Apricots, dried	4 halves
Banana	½ small
Blackberries and blueberries	½ cup
Boysenberries	⅔ cup
Cantaloupe	¾ cup
Cherries, fresh or canned	10 large
Dates	2 small
Figs	1 large
Grapefruit	½ small
Grapes	12
Guava	1 small
Honeydew	⅛ cup
Kumquat	3–4 medium
Loganberries	½ cup

Mango	½ small
Nectarine	1 medium
Orange	1 small
Papaya	⅓ medium
Peach	1 medium
Pear	1 small
Pineapple	½ cup
Pineapple ring (canned)	1
Plums	2 medium
Pomegranate	1 small
Prunes	2 medium
Raisins	2 tbsp
Raspberries	½ cup
Strawberries	1 cup
Tangerine	2 small
Watermelon	1 cup

Exchanges are for fresh or frozen fruit or those canned without added sugar.

Orange juice	½ cup
Grapefruit juice	½ cup
Pineapple juice	⅓ cup
Prune juice	¼ cup

Bread, Cereals, and Starchy Vegetables

For each bread exchange on your food plan, you may choose one of the following. Remember that while all whole-grain and enriched cereals are good sources of B vitamins and iron, whole-wheat, rye, and whole-grain cereals are better foods than refined cereals because they contain more fiber.

BREADS

Bagel	½
Biscuits (baking powder)	1
Slice of bread	1

Bread crumbs	1 cup
Bread sticks (4 to 6 inches)	4
Cornbread (plus 1 fat exchange)*	1
Hamburger bun (medium)	1
Hot-dog bun	1
Melba toast	4
Blueberry muffin (plus 1 fat exchange)	1
Bran muffin (plus 1 fat exchange)	1
English muffin	½
Pancakes (4-inch diameter) (plus 1 fat exchange)	1
Raisin bread (slice)	1
Roll	1
Rusk	2
Taco or tostada shell	1
Tortilla	1
Waffle (plus 1 fat exchange)	1
Zwieback	3

CEREALS

All-bran	⅓ cup
Barley (cooked)	½ cup
Barley (uncooked)	1 tbsp
Cooked cereal	½ cup
Flaked or puffed cold cereal	¾ cup
Grapenuts	3 tbsp
Grapenut flakes	½ cup
Grits	½ cup
Raisin bran	½ cup
Shredded wheat biscuit	1
Wheat germ	2 tbsp

CRACKERS

Graham (2½-inch square)	2
Matzo (6-inch diameter)	1

*Note that when breads are made with substantial quantities of fat, the fat must be taken into consideration when exchanging.

Tea matzo (2½-inch square, thin) 5
Oyster 20
Pretzel (twisted medium) 6
Thin pretzels (stick) 20
Round thin pretzel (plus 1 fat exchange) 6
Saltine (2-inch square) 5

POTATO, RICE, AND PASTA

White potato (the size of an egg) 1
White potato, mashed .... ½ cup
Sweet potato or yam .... ¼ cup
Rice (cooked) .... ½ cup
Pasta, noodles, spaghetti, etc. .... ½ cup

STARCHY VEGETABLES

Dried lima, navy, pinto beans; split peas and
chickpeas .... ½ cup
Baked beans (no pork) .... ¼ cup
Baked beans (with pork and molasses; plus 1 fat
exchange) .... 3 tbsp
Corn .... ⅓ cup
Corn on the cob 1
Hominy .... ½ cup
Mixed vegetables .... ½ cup
Parsnips .... ⅔ cup
Green peas .... ½ cup
Popcorn (if coated with butter, add 1 fat
exchange) .... 1½ cups
Pumpkin .... ¾ cup
Squash: winter, acorn, and butternut .... ½ cup

DESSERTS

Arrowroot cookies 3
Animal cookies (plain) 8
Fig Newton bar 1
Gingerbread (1″ × 1″ × 2″) 1

Gingersnaps .... 4 small
Vanilla wafers 5
Ice cream (plus 2 fat exchanges) .... ½ cup

Meat, Fish, Poultry, Eggs, and Cheese (also Peanut Butter)

These are the main protein foods in all but vegetarian food plans. Roast, broil, boil, and stew meats rather than frying them for everyday use. Save the frying for special occasions. Then, be sure to include the frying fat in your fat exchanges for that meal. Trim off all visible fat before cooking. A 4-ounce portion of raw meat is the same as a 3-ounce portion of cooked meat. Meat is divided into lean, medium, and high-fat. Serve high-fat meats only occasionally.

Lean Meat

Each ounce of lean meat contains approximately 7 grams of protein, 2.5 grams of fat, and about 50 calories.

Any fresh or frozen fish .... 1 ounce
Canned salmon, tuna, mackerel, crab .... ¼ cup
Lobster (canned) .... ¼ cup
Sardines (drained) .... 3 each
Clams, oysters, scallops, shrimp 5
Textured vegetable protein (plus 1 bread
exchange) .... 2 tbsp
Peanut butter (plus 2 fat exchanges) .... 2 tbsp
Poultry (chicken, turkey, etc., without skin) ...... 1 ounce
Pork (leg, whole rump, smoked ham,
organ meat) .... 1 ounce
Veal (all cuts except breast) .... 1 ounce
Beef: baby beef, chipped beef, chuck, flank,
tenderloin, plate ribs, plate skirt, round,
sirloin tip, rump, spare ribs, tripe,
organ meats .... 1 ounce

Lamb leg, rib, sirloin, loin, shank, shoulder ...... 1 ounce
Lamb organ meats .... 1 ounce
Cheese (less than 5 percent butterfat) .... 1 ounce
Cottage cheese (low-fat) .... ¼ cup

MEDIUM-FAT MEAT

Each ounce of medium-fat meat contains 7 grams of protein, 5 grams of fat, and 73 calories.

Soybean curd (tofu) .... ½ cup
Egg 1
Pork loin (all cuts), tenderloin, shoulder, arm,
picnic, shoulder blade, Canadian bacon,
boiled ham, picnic ham (loin or
shoulder) .... 1 ounce
Beef: ground beef (15 percent fat), ground round,
corned beef (canned), rib eye, sirloin .... 1 ounce
Cheese: cottage cheese (creamed) .... ¼ cup
edam, mozzarella, ricotta, farmer .... 1 ounce
parmesan .... 3 tbsp

HIGH-FAT MEAT

Each ounce of high-fat meat contains 7 grams of protein, 7.5 grams of fat, and 95 calories.

Poultry (capon, goose, duck) .... 1 ounce
Pork spareribs, ground pork, country-style ham .. 1 ounce
sausage and pork links (plus 2 fat
exchanges) 2
Veal breast .... 1 ounce
Beef brisket (fresh and corned), ground beef
(more than 20 percent fat), hamburger
(commercial), rib roast, club and rib
steaks .... 1 ounce
Lamb breast .... 1 ounce

Cold cuts .... 1 ounce
Frankfurter 1
Cheese: cheddar type, American, Roquefort,
Gruyère, Limburger, Swiss, Liederkranz .... 1 ounce

Fats

All fats have many calories. Fats are divided into three groups: polyunsaturated, monosaturated, and saturated. Polyunsaturated fats are generally liquid at room temperature. Most saturated fats are solid. It is best for everyone to avoid saturated fats as much as possible. This advice is doubly important for those with diabetes, even children.

Polyunsaturated fats

Margarine (with liquid polyunsaturated oil listed
as first ingredient on package) .... 1 tsp
Diet margarine (with liquid polyunsaturated oil
listed as first ingredient on package) .... 2 tsp
Nuts
Almonds 8
Filberts 5
Hickory 7
Pecans 3
Chopped pecans .... 1 tbsp
Pistachios 20
Sunflower seeds .... 1½ tbsp
Walnuts (whole) 3
Chopped walnuts .... 1½ tbsp
Oils (in descending order of polyunsaturation)
Safflower .... 1 tsp
Corn .... 1 tsp
Soybean .... 1 tsp
Sunflower .... 1 tsp
Cottonseed .... 1 tsp
Sesame .... 1 tsp

Salad Dressings

Creamy dressing (made from package with 1 part buttermilk, 1 part mayonnaise) .... 2 tsp
(made with 1 part buttermilk, 1 part imitation mayonnaise) .... 4 tsp
(made with 1 part buttermilk, 1 part imitation sour cream) .... 3 tbsp
French dressing .... 1 tbsp
Italian dressing .... 1 tbsp
Mayonnaise (regular) .... 1 tsp
Mayonnaise (imitation) .... 2 tsp
Salad dressing (mayonnaise type) .... 2 tsp
Thousand Island dressing .... 2 tsp
Cream substitute (made from polyunsaturated oil) .... 2 tbsp
Sour cream substitute (made from polyunsaturated oil) .... 2 tbsp
Tartar sauce .... 2 tsp

Monosaturated Fats

Avocado (4-inch diameter) 1/8
Slice of crisp bacon 1
Brazil nuts 2
Peanuts 6
Green olives 3
Ripe olives 5
Olive oil .... 1 tsp
Peanut oil .... 1 tsp

Saturated Fats

These foods should be reserved for special treats.
Butter .... 1 tsp
Chocolate (unsweetened) .... 2 tsp
Coconut (fresh 1 × 1 × 1½-inch) .... 1 piece
Coconut oil .... 1 tsp

Cream cheese .... 1 tbsp
Cream (heavy) .... 2 tbsp
Cream (half and half) .... 2 tbsp
Sour cream .... 2 tbsp
Cashew nuts 6
Macadamia nuts 3
Blue cheese salad dressing .... 2 tsp

Free List

These foods may be used as desired, as they contain little if any carbohydrates, protein, and fat.

Beverages
Broth
Bouillon
Club soda
Coffee
Tea
Postum
Sugar-free soft drinks
Low-calorie salad dressing (limit to reasonable amount)
Condiments
Sauces like catsup, soy sauce, taco sauce, etc. ... 1 tbsp

Flavorings such as celery powder, flavor extracts, garlic, ginger, herbs, mint, parsley, spices, gelatin, pectin, cranberries (unsweetened), lemon, sugar substitutes, rhubarb.

Q: *How do I use this information to create a meal plan?*
A: Let us suppose that the dietician recommends that your child's breakfast consist of 3 bread exchanges, 2 fat exchanges, 1 fruit exchange, and 1 milk exchange. You might use any of these menus:

BREAKFAST MENU #1

1 fresh orange juice .... 1 fruit exchange
¾ cup cornflakes .... 1 bread exchange
1 cup milk (some poured over cereal) . 1 milk exchange
1 toasted English muffin .... 2 bread exchanges plus 1 fat exchange
1 tsp margarine .... 1 fat exchange

BREAKFAST MENU #2

1 fresh orange, sliced .... 1 fruit exchange
2 pancakes with wheat germ .... 3 bread exchanges plus 1 fat exchange
1 slice bacon .... 1 fat exchange
8 ounces of milk .... 1 milk exchange

BREAKFAST MENU #3

½ cup oatmeal sprinkled with 2 tbsp raisins and 1 tbsp cream .... 1 bread exchange, 1 fruit exchange, and 1 fat exchange
2 slices whole-wheat bread .... 2 bread exchanges
1 tsp margarine .... 1 fat exchange
8 ounces milk .... 1 milk exchange

BREAKFAST MENU #4

grapefruit sections with avocado ...... 1 fruit exchange plus 1 fat exchange
¾ cup puffed rice cereal .... 1 bread exchange
1 bagel with cream cheese .... 2 bread plus 1 fat exchange
8 ounces milk .... 1 milk exchange

All these menus contain the same number of exchanges, yet some are more nutritious than others. Menu 1 and menu 4 have less fiber (note fruit-juice rather than whole fruit and cereals and breads made from refined flour). All are within the guidelines, yet your family would be better nourished with the foods in menus

2 and 3. There is no need to do this all at once. Small substitutions will hardly be noticed by the family, and they can be weaned away from food high in sugars, fats, and salt gradually and quietly.

Q: *Does that mean that we shouldn't eat a cooked breakfast of bacon, eggs, and sausages anymore?*
A: Eat it if you enjoy it, but don't eat it every day. Make it a special treat for Sundays and holidays. You will enjoy it even more because it is a treat. And try serving the eggs scrambled in a nonstick pan, coddled, or poached instead of fried in bacon grease. You might also try an egg substitute. Grill the bacon and the sausages instead of frying them. Use only a scraping of margarine on your toast. Talk to your dietician about how to borrow fat and meat exchanges from other meals that day for your bacon and egg breakfast.

Q: *What about jam and jelly? Should I get diabetic ones?*
A: If the amount of jam or jelly used is small—say, a teaspoonful on bread with a meal—it hardly matters. If your child is very fond of them and uses large quantities on his bread or for peanut-butter-and-jelly sandwiches, then a sugarless kind is in order.

Q: *What about other diabetic foods?*
A: I wouldn't bother with most of them. Generally, they are substitutions for very sweet foods that have little food value. It is better to work toward coaxing the family away from these foods into healthier eating patterns than to reproduce the old habits using sugar substitutes. They can come in handy at times, though. If you are in the habit of distributing candy to your children regularly, you can give a diabetic candy to your child with diabetes at these times. It is far better, though, to give all your children fresh and dried fruits, nuts, seeds, popcorn, and other sugarless treats than to get them used to large amounts of sugar, which causes tooth decay, poor appetite, and can lead to other health problems in the future.

Q: *What about drinks?*
A: Milk and fresh fruit juices have more food value than fruitades, whether sugar-free or full of sugar. Fruitades are no more than sweetened colored water, and even the coloring agents are harmful to some children who are sensitive to the chemicals used. If your children are accustomed to drinking large amounts of these beverages, try making your own from fruit juice and water. The addition of ice and a good dollop of club or sugar-free soda plus some lemon or lime slices make these very attractive. Be careful to keep the mix weak. Fruit juice will elevate the blood glucose quickly, and these punches should contain only enough fruit juice to flavor them. There are sugar-free sodas in every conceivable flavor, but a better option for your children is mineral water, still or sparkling, which is refreshing and encourages better health habits.

Q: *What about desserts? My child loves desserts and would feel deprived without them. Are there special diabetic desserts on the market?*
A: There are all sorts of diabetic gelatin and milk-pudding desserts in your supermarket that taste the same as the nondiabetic variety except that they are made with a sugar substitute. I often make gelatin desserts at home, though, as they are much tastier. You can drain the juice from a can of fruit (make sure that it is canned in juice, not syrup) and add gelatin. When the mixture is half set, add the fruit. A dollop of whipped cream (low-fat variety) makes an attractive family dessert. You can also use vanilla ice cream with a few strawberries or a banana slice on the top garnished with a spray of low-fat whipped cream. With a bit of thought, almost any dessert can be made from ingredients that are reduced in sugar and fat. Half a peach or pear (fresh or canned in fruit juice) in which is nestling a small scoop of vanilla ice cream with a shaving of diabetic chocolate (grated with a cheese grater) looks quite attractive and should satisfy any child's yearning for a special dessert.

Q: *What about apple pie a la mode, my family's favorite?*
A: If you bake the pie yourself using whole-grain flour and fresh apples rather than white flour and canned apples, you will immediately improve the fiber content and reduce the sugar. You can sweeten the apples with saccharin or aspartame (Sugar-Twin and Sweet 'N Low are saccharins, Equal and NutraSweet are aspartames). The ice cream should be vanilla. If you have an ice-cream maker, this can be reduced in fat and sugar as well, because you can make your own. If not, there are many varieties of low-fat ice cream or ice milk in the supermarket. However, desserts like this should not be everyday fare. They are for serving as special treats for holiday dinners. A piece of fresh fruit is a healthier dessert for everyday eating. If you save all the sweet foods for one particular day, say Sunday, you can increase the insulin dose slightly on that day to cover them.

Q: *Is there a healthier substitute for cream? My family likes cream with every dessert from fruit to cake.*
A: Try low-fat yogurt, plain or fruit-flavored, as a topping for desserts. Plain yogurt is delicious on a baked apple or with berries. Don't make an issue of these things, but try to increase the variety of your family's diet gradually by offering foods that look attractive and are similar to the old favorites.

Q: *Is yogurt a permitted food for persons with diabetes?*
A: Yes. One cup of yogurt made from low-fat milk is 1 milk exchange and 1 fat exchange. The fruit-flavored varieties should be sweetened with an artificial sweetener. The tart taste of plain yogurt is a perfect foil for fruit, just as nice as sour cream or sweet cream. In fact, you will find that once you begin to cut down on sugar in your diet, your taste buds will sharpen and other foods will taste better to you. After a time, you will detect even some of the sugar hidden in processed foods that you never noticed before.

Q: *I have heard persons with diabetes talk about fruit sugar. What is fruit sugar and how is it different from other sugars?*
A: The sugar in the usual bag in the supermarket is sucrose. It is made from sugarcane or beet, processed and refined. Fruit sugar, or fructose, is the natural sugar found in fruit. It can also be processed and refined. It is twice as sweet as sucrose, so that only half the amount is required. It has been shown that people with diabetes can tolerate fructose better than sucrose. Small amounts do not cause the marked rise in blood glucose that is evident after eating sucrose. Still, doctors recommend only 2 ounces a day. Use it sparingly in cooking. It is quite expensive compared with sucrose. I recommend its use on special occasions only. For everyday living, try to eat fewer sugary foods.

The foods that are essential to good health are fresh fruit and vegetables, dairy products, cereals including bread, rice, and pasta, and meat, fish, and poultry along with some oils. Vegetarians eat more vegetable protein to make up for eating no animal protein. None of these foods contains sugar. The sugar you buy in a sack is a completely unnecessary food. If you never bought another ounce of it, your health would not suffer. In fact, there is good evidence that it would improve. So consider all food made from sugar as extra to your basic food needs—pleasant for special occasions but not essential to good nutrition.

Q: *What about artificial sweeteners? Are they safe?*
A: The Food and Drug Administration has studied this issue carefully and come up with guidelines for the use of artificial sweeteners. There are two types of sugar substitutes now on the market: saccharin and aspartame. Saccharin is the sweetening agent in Sweet 'N Low and Sugar Twin; aspartame is the sweetening agent in Equal and NutraSweet.

The FDA has established the following safety levels for these products. Saccharin: for children, 500 mg per day (20 to 30 packets, each containing 1 teaspoonful). Double that amount may be used by adults. Aspartame: 23 mg per pound of body weight. For a child weighing 75 pounds, that is the amount used to sweeten eight 12-ounce cans of soft drink. An adult weighing 154 pounds can consume 17 cans and still be within the limit.

Q: *My child likes to sprinkle sugar on his morning cereal. What kind of sweetener is best?*
A: Don't use fruit sugar. Fructose on its own is too sweet for such purposes. It is better saved for cooking. Some people use small amounts of aspartame sweeteners, but I don't really recommend them for this purpose. Breakfast cereals don't need to be sweet. It is only a bad habit. Try slices of fresh or canned fruit as a substitute. Try raisins or currants. Or you might try a different breakfast until he stops yearning for sugared cereal. Pancakes using whole-meal flour and buttermilk or plain yogurt are lovely, and if you mix all the dry ingredients beforehand, you need to add only the milk, egg, and butter or margarine to the mixture in the morning. It takes only a few minutes to mix the batter and drop it by the spoonful onto a greased griddle or frying pan. These pancakes can be served with diabetic jam or jelly. A plateful with a fresh orange and a glass of milk makes a nutritious breakfast or supper for any child. (Make sure that you add a teaspoon of baking soda to the mix if you use buttermilk or yogurt.)

If you have a waffle iron (some sandwich makers have waffle plates, too), you can use the same batter to cook waffles. These waffles are far superior to the frozen commercial waffles and have no added sugar. If you have the time, you can bake stacks of them and freeze them. Then your child can reheat them in the toaster and serve them to his friends just like the ready-made ones. It is important that your child be able to entertain his friends in exactly the same way that he would do if he did not have diabetes. Making him different will always be detrimental to him.

Q: *Can you recommend any other treats that my diabetic child can fix by himself?*
A: He can make an ice-cream soda by putting a scoop of ice cream into a tall glass and topping it up with sugar-free soda. Just

stir until foamy. Serve with a straw and a long spoon. This is guaranteed to delight any young child, and is a standby of mine for birthday parties.

Q: *What is the best thing to do for birthday parties? The food served is very sweet.*

A: With my own child, I found that the best thing to do was nothing. I let her enjoy herself. Birthday parties are rare occasions. The children expend so much energy running around playing that the excess carbohydrates are soon used up. For the parties that you give yourself, you can tailor the menu to suit your own ideas. For example, the cake does not have to be frosted with sugar. Use either a sugar-free frosting mix or put vanilla ice cream on the top. Sugar-free soda is readily available or, better yet, if you have a punch bowl or large pitcher, a pretty punch can be made from fresh juices, club soda, ice, and fruit.

If you feel that you must distribute candy, save it for going home. That way, the other children will be eating their chocolate bars on the way home and not in front of your youngster. Serve little bowls of nuts, pretzels, and popcorn at the party. Grapes and other small fruits are nice too. However, if your child protests against any changes in the traditional party menu, don't worry. His birthday comes only once a year, and the birthday child is usually too excited to eat much anyway.

Q: *What about holidays with special foods, like Christmas or Passover?*

A: You'll find that the diabetes magazines are chock-full of recipes suitable for Christmas cooking. Diabetic cookbooks have them as well. As far as Passover is concerned, the problem is not so much sugar as fat. You can try various fat substitutes, especially for chicken fat. But then again, who can really enjoy chopped liver without a bit of schmaltz!

Fortunately, these holidays come only once a year, and if small portions of the suspect foods are given, I do not believe that any lasting harm will be done. Holiday menus are usually planned in advance, often for weeks, even months, so you can increase the insulin dose slightly on these occasions. If you allow sweet treats with a meal rather than as between-meal snacks, they will not cause blood-glucose levels to rise as much. Don't worry about this. With a bit of experience, you will know when to allow certain foods and when to offer sugarless substitutes. There will be many times when your child's blood glucose will be low and you will be able to reach into the goody box for a special treat. The important thing to remember when your child is diagnosed is that diabetes is for life. Giving the child too many restrictions will only make him rebellious, and rebellion is the state that you want to avoid at all costs. Better to have the odd fluctuation in control than for him to turn against his condition in adolescence and refuse to look after himself.

Remember also that forbidden fruit is always sweeter. If you make a habit of hiding cakes and candy to be eaten by others when he is not around, you are only storing up problems for him in the future. If your child catches a glimpse of something he wants, give him a small piece and say nothing. If it is extremely sweet, tell him that it is being saved for dinner and give him a tiny piece then, when it will do less harm. Don't underline his condition by saying, as I have heard many mothers say, "You can only have a little portion, because you have diabetes." Give all the children little portions and answer any complaints by telling them that too much sugar is bad for their teeth. After a while, you will find that it is easier to keep these things out of the house and you will all get used to eating less sugar.

Q: *My child's food plan, given to us in the hospital, says that the only permissible dessert is fresh fruit or plain yogurt. Jam, jelly, candy, and cake are forbidden. Isn't this right?*

A: Your child's food plan is a guide for you both. It is not the gospel. Human beings are complex and far from perfect. Compromise is necessary in all human relations. There is a psychological element in all physical illness. An unhappy child is going to be more difficult to control. It is better to yield a little at times on these rules than to insist on perfection and push your child into rebelling against the diabetic regime.

Q: *My child is used to sitting in the grocery cart and getting a candy bar at the checkout. How can I cope with this now that he has diabetes?*
A: There are several ways to handle this situation. You could leave him at home or with a friend instead of taking him to the supermarket. You could substitute sugar-free chewing gum (usually sold at the checkout as well) or keep a piece of diabetic candy in your bag for such occasions. You might divert him by offering a piece of fruit, bag of nuts, or a package of popcorn instead. Don't be bullied. This problem usually arises because there are long lines at the checkout and the child gets bored and restless. Perhaps bringing a toy or small game would help. Could you shop at an hour when the store is less crowded? Many supermarkets are open late at night.

Q: *Can my child eat the school lunch, or should I provide a brown-bag lunch for him?*
A: Either choice is appropriate. It is the content of the meal that is important, not whether it comes from your kitchen or the school's. If the child enjoys eating the school lunch, let him. There is usually more involved than the actual eating of the meal. Often, the choice of whether to bring a brown-bag lunch or not has social ramifications. The children divide themselves up at lunch time, sit with certain friends, spend a certain amount of time in the schoolyard or doing their homework. These patterns establish themselves early in the term. Changing from one option to another in the middle of the term might be upsetting. If he is used to eating the school lunch, it would be better to check that the meal is suitable, make any changes necessary, and then let him go on as usual.

Q: *How can I decide whether or not the school meals are suitable?*
A: Get a list of menus from the principal. If you cannot estimate the number of exchanges yourself yet, ask your dietician to help you. This is a problem that dieticians deal with all the time. You will probably find that the school lunch is more than sufficient for your child's midday meal. Undoubtedly, the dessert is too sweet and rich, but the rest of the lunch will fit into his food plan. In that case, if your child can be trusted to substitute fresh fruit or a diet yogurt for the dessert, give him some to take with him. If you think that the temptation to eat the dessert will be more than he can resist, you can speak to the school authorities about substituting a more suitable dessert for him. However, you should discuss the matter with your child. If he is old enough to stay in school for the lunch hour, he is old enough to have a preference. Be tactful. Try to arrive at a mutually agreeable solution. This will avoid the situation where the child eats the school dessert surreptitiously, setting a pattern for future deception and promoting the consumption of unsuitable food to an act of defiance against his parents.

Also, it is important to prevent the school staff, in a misguided attempt to be helpful, to embarrass your child by making an issue of the fact that he has to eat special food. He doesn't, and they shouldn't think that he does. I have heard tales of an overzealous teacher who snatched a dish of ice cream from under the nose of a child, crying, "You can't have that, you have diabetes," and of one who herded several children together at a separate table, shouting at them as they entered the room, "Diabetics, this way!" This kind of well-meaning but tactless behavior can hurt your child's feelings. Diabetes is a blow to him. Having to do shots is a trauma. You don't want to inflict an additional burden by making him feel different.

Q: *If I give my child a brown-bag lunch, what shall I pack?*
A: First, you must look at the meal plan that he has received

from the dietician or the doctor. How many exchanges does it recommend? How are they divided? Let us suppose that your child is to eat 2 bread exchanges, 1 milk exchange, 2 fruit exchanges, 1 vegetable exchange, 2 meat exchanges, and 1 fat exchange. You might create menus like these:

BROWN-BAG LUNCH #1

Sandwich made from 2 slices of white bread filled with egg salad, canned fish, cheese, peanut butter, sliced meat, etc. This contains

2 bread exchanges, 2 meat exchanges, 1 fat exchange

1 piece of fruit .... 1 fruit exchange
salad of grated carrots and raisins .. 1 veg exchange, 1 fruit
1 small diet yogurt .... 1 milk exchange
can of diet soda .... free

BROWN-BAG LUNCH #2

Sandwich made from 2 slices whole-wheat, rye, or pumpernickel bread filled with egg salad, canned fish, cheese, peanut butter, sliced meat, etc. This contains

2 bread exchanges, 2 meat exchanges, 1 fat exchange

salad of lettuce, celery, and apple
segments dressed with lemon
juice .... 1 veg exchange, 1 fruit
cup of milk .... 1 milk exchange

BROWN-BAG LUNCH #3

Thermos of vegetable soup .... 1 vegetable exchange
2 slices cornbread .... 2 bread exchanges
plus 1 fat exchange
small box cottage cheese .... 2 meat exchanges
banana .... 2 fruit exchanges
cup of milk .... 1 milk exchange

BROWN-BAG LUNCH #4

Thermos of stew with meat, vegetable, lentils	2 meat exchanges, 1 vegetable exchange, 1 bread exchange
salad of grated raw vegetables with small amount dressing	1 vegetable exchange, ½ fat exchange
peach	1 fruit exchange
8 animal cookies	1 bread exchange
small diet yogurt	1 milk exchange, ½ fat exchange
diet soda	free

You can see how easy it is to fashion menus that suit your child's taste from the myriad of nourishing foods available. All these sample menus have the same number of exchanges, but menus 3 and 4 include a hot dish and menu 2 is preferable to menu 1 because of the choice of bread.

Q: *What about a snack at recess time?*
A: It is fortunate that all schools allow time for between-meal snacks so that your child's need for frequent meals can easily be catered to. Most elementary schools provide milk and cookies midmorning. If the cookies are not too sweet, let your child eat one with the others. If you think the cookie unsuitable, speak quietly to the teacher. Perhaps you can provide a box of graham crackers or arrowroot cookies for your child. It would be better, of course, if you sent enough for all the children.

Q: *What about snacks out of the classroom—in the schoolyard, for example—where each child provides his own? Most of the children eat candy at this time.*
A: If the others eat candy, provide your child with a package of diabetic candy, but be sure to add a piece of fruit or a package

of low-fat potato chips or pretzels so that he gets some carbohydrates.

Q: *Does he need an afternoon snack as well as a morning one?*
A: Yes. He needs to eat something every two and a half to three hours. However, most children do this anyway. If you live near the school, he can come straight home and have his afternoon snack at home. If he has to travel home by bus or if he stays in school to play or for any after-school activity, he should take his snack with him.

Q: *What sort of food is best?*
A: Consult your food plan. If he is allowed 1 bread exchange and 1 milk or fruit exchange, the following would be appropriate: milk and cookie, milk and sandwich, apple and popcorn, or plain cake and low-fat, sugarless cocoa.

Q: *Most of my child's friends buy ice Pops on the way home from school. What do I do about this?*
A: Make your own ice Pops from fruit juice or punch sweetened with sugar substitutes. Let him have one of these after school, but make sure that he takes something substantial with it. Starchy foods that take longer to be digested are better afternoon snacks. If you can, save the ice Pops for dessert.

Q: *What sort of foods are suitable for dinner?*
A: If the evening meal is dinner for the whole family, the usual combination of meat, vegetables, and potatoes (or pasta or rice) with fruit or a simple dessert is as suitable for him as for the other members of the family. This meal is entirely under your control, so you can make the most of it as a time to introduce healthier eating habits. Try serving fish and poultry more often than meat, and increase the amount and variety of fresh vegetables, lightly cooked or raw. Small children usually love raw carrot sticks or celery stalks. Encourage this. If your family insists on fried chicken with french fries, drain the potatoes well on paper towels or in

clean paper bags. Cut them thick. Thin ones absorb more grease. Don't re-use the oil. With each lot you fry, the oil becomes more saturated. Fry the chicken only until it is golden brown. Then place the pieces on a wire rack over a baking tin and put into a moderate oven for 30 to 40 minutes. The chicken can finish cooking there, allowing some of the oil to drain away. Make fried chicken with all the trimmings a special treat for someone's birthday or a holiday. Everyday dinners should make more use of baked, boiled, and mashed potatoes (use low-fat margarine rather than butter for mashing them. No one will ever taste the difference). If you think about each of the family's favorite foods in turn, you will be able to substitute healthier ingredients or different cooking methods for almost all dishes, which will make them more nutritious. For example, bread crumbs and stuffing can be made from whole-grain breads instead of white. Low-fat milk tastes little different from full-cream once you get used to it. Coleslaw can be dressed with safflower oil and cider vinegar instead of mayonnaise. Berries can be topped with low-fat yogurt instead of sour cream. Ice milk can be substituted for ice cream. Sugar substitutes can be used in cooking and baking. Rhubarb or applesauce taste just as good sweetened with saccharin or aspartame as with sugar. Pie crusts can be made with whole-wheat flour. The list is endless. You can be as creative and imaginative as you like.

Q: *Can you suggest a few dinner menus that incorporate these ideas and show me how to count the exchanges in them?*
A: Here are a few simple menus incorporating old ideas and new. The exchanges are shown for each serving.

MENU #1

clear soup or bouillon .... free
4 ounces roast chicken with
  skin removed .... 4 lean meat exchanges
natural gravy .... negligible
baked potato (6 ounces or the size
  of 3 eggs) .... 3 bread exchanges

butter beans .... 1 bread exchange
lettuce and tomato salad .... 2 vegetable exchanges
8 ounces milk .... 1 milk exchange
fresh fruit cocktail with 2 tbsp
plain low-fat yogurt .... 1 fruit exchange
plus ½ milk exchange
and ¼ fat exchange

MENU #2

lentil and vegetable soup .... 1 bread exchange,
1 vegetable exchange,
½ fat exchange
cheese omelette .... 3 medium-fat meat
exchanges per serving
french fries .... 2 bread and
1½ fat exchanges
baked beans (vegetarian) .... 1 bread exchange
8 ounces milk .... 1 milk exchange
sugarless gelatin dessert .... ½ fruit exchange

MENU #3

fresh vegetable salad with
oil-and-vinegar dressing .... 2 vegetable exchanges,
1 fat exchange
spaghetti with meatballs .... 3 medium-fat meat
exchanges,
3 bread exchanges,
1 vegetable exchange,
½ fat exchange
1 slice garlic bread .... 1 bread exchange,
½ fat exchange
vanilla ice milk sprinkled with
walnuts .... 1 milk exchange,
2 fat exchanges
diet drink .... free

MENU #4

¼ lb hamburger with roll .... 4 medium-fat exchanges, 1 bread exchange

french fries .... 3 bread exchanges, 1½ fat exchanges

coleslaw with diet mayonnaise dressing .... 1 vegetable exchange, 2 fat exchanges

milkshake made with low-fat milk, ice milk .... 1 milk exchange, ½ bread exchange, 1 fat exchange

MENU #5

½ grapefruit .... 1 fruit exchange

grilled fish (6 ounces) .... 6 lean meat exchanges

mashed potato .... 3 bread exchanges, 1 fat exchange, negligible milk

steamed broccoli .... 1 vegetable exchange

corn on cob .... 1 bread exchange

sugar-free chocolate pudding ..... 1 milk exchange, ½ fat exchange

cup of milk .... 1 milk exchange

MENU #6

shrimp cocktail .... 1 lean meat exchange, 1 fat exchange for dressing

broiled sirloin steak (4 ounces) ... 4 medium-fat meat exchanges

baked potato with 2 tbsp plain yogurt .... 3 bread exchanges, ¼ milk exchange, ¼ fat exchange

green peas .... 1 bread exchange
fresh vegetable salad with low-cal
dressing .... 2 vegetable exchanges, ½ fat exchange
strawberries .... 1 fruit exchange
milk .... 1 milk exchange

All these menus have approximately 40 grams of carbohydrate, although they are divided among different foods. None of the dinners given here is anything but ordinary American food, available in any supermarket and using common cooking skills. They are probably similar to the foods you have been serving your family for years.

Q: *What foods have to be eliminated altogether?*
A: None. All foods have their place, even candy. I have found that the easiest way to handle requests for inappropriate foods is to suggest that they be saved for another time. If your child's diabetes is carefully controlled, there will be many times when his blood glucose will be low and sugar is required to bring it up to normal. He should carry something sweet in his pocket for these occasions.

Q: *How can I be certain that the candy in his pocket won't find its way into his mouth at the wrong time?*
A: The only way that you can be reasonably certain of this is by discussing it with your child. Unless he is very young, he can be taught about food values. His desire to cheat is usually fueled by his normal and natural need to assert his independence. If you allow him as much independence as is appropriate for a child of his age, he will be less likely to sneak inappropriate foods in order to feel grown-up. It is also a good idea to stop buying these foods. It is grossly unfair as well as unrealistic to forbid a child to help himself to sugary cookies when the kitchen cupboards are overflowing with them. If you enjoy cooking, bake these things at

home. You can use more healthful ingredients and less sugar if you do. If cooking is not your strong suit or if your time in the kitchen is limited, perhaps there is someone else in the family or among your friends who enjoys cooking and would be pleased to bake for you. Often, a grandmother is only too delighted to be called upon in this regard. In addition to the obvious benefits of having a supply of home-baked food, there is also a great psychological boost from sharing this problem. Looking after a child with diabetes is very taxing emotionally. There seems to be no respite from worry. There is much to be gained from involving another adult in this concern. A good diabetic cookbook (there are many on the market) would help this person to adapt her recipes to suit your child's needs.

Q: *Somebody told me that her dietician forbids all canned and packaged soups. I don't have the time to cook soup. What can I do?*
A: The first thing you can do is to stop listening to everyone's advice. If you don't, you will end up hemmed in by hundreds of prohibitions and misconceptions. There are many different types of commercial soups. Some are clear, bouillons and consommés that have very little food value but that might have quite a lot of added sugar. If the second ingredient on the label is sugar, you can be certain that the sugar content is high and the food value low. You would probably not be giving these to your children anyway. Soups with vegetables and meat have varying food values. Ask your dietician for a list of those commercial soups that can be used fairly freely, but also think again about making your own. The soups you remember from your childhood, the soups your mother or grandmother made, were probably tastier, free from additives such as taste boosters and coloring agents, and were less expensive. I think that your friend's dietician was urging her to use less convenience food. This is certainly a good idea. It really takes very little time to cook a large pot of soup once or twice a week. It is an economical way of using leftovers and it also ensures that

your family gets plenty of fresh vegetables, especially if yours is a family that doesn't like vegetables other than frozen peas or baked beans.

Q: *Are all convenience foods to be omitted?*
A: It is hard to make general rules that apply to everyone. Convenience foods have multiplied enormously in the past twenty years, due in part to the fact that fewer women are full-time homemakers now. Avoiding all convenience foods is impossible. But many people who have the time to cook and who enjoy cooking have fallen into the habit of using convenience foods and ready-cooked foods just because they are there, arrayed temptingly on the supermarket shelves or in the freezers. Next time you shop for food, take a critical look at your cart before you reach the check-out. Do you really need to buy that frozen pie? What happened to the delicious pies you used to bake? Are those frozen and canned vegetables good value? Fresh vegetables in season are tastier and have a nicer texture. Read labels carefully. You will be amazed to learn how many manufactured foods are full of water and chemicals. To answer your question simply, use convenience foods if you have to, but try to incorporate more fresh foods and homemade dishes into your family's eating plan. That way, you will know precisely what you are serving them.

Q: *Does my child need a bedtime snack?*
A: Yes. It is normal for blood-glucose levels to fall during the night, reach their lowest levels during the early hours of the morning, and then rise slowly as the day dawns. The bedtime snack should be one that will be digested slowly so that its energy will be released during the time when blood sugars are low. Cereal or bread are good choices. Your child might like a sandwich or a bowl of cold cereal with milk and banana slices.

Q: *What about cocoa?*
A: Milky drinks are fine so long as they are accompanied by a bread exchange to slow down absorption. Make certain, however,

that you choose a brand made with an artificial sweetener. Some cocoas are reduced in calories for dieters. These would be reduced in fat as well as sugar.

Q: *What do you think of a diabetic chocolate Santa Claus or Easter egg?*
A: Check the labels. These particular candies are often sweetened with sorbitol. Large amounts of sorbitol can cause diarrhea and stomachaches. If small pieces are eaten at a time, there is no harm in them. If, however, your child will devour the entire confection at one sitting, he will probably get more sorbitol than is wise. One Christmas product that is more manageable than a chocolate Santa Claus is a little bag of chocolate coins wrapped in gold paper. You can put a few of these into his Christmas stocking and give one or two a day over the holiday period when the other children are being given gifts of chocolate.

Q: *What about other types of diabetic chocolate? Are they all sweetened with sorbitol?*
A: Many are sweetened with fructose. These are quite nice and taste more like ordinary chocolate. They are useful for grating over desserts, too. Generally, however, I would regard these candies as special treats and not offer them too often. Watermelon, cherries, fresh apricots, mangoes, strawberries, etc., are better choices and even more delicious.

Q: *What about alcohol? I like to cook with wine sometimes.*
A: When you heat wine, the alcohol virtually disappears. Only the taste remains. Besides, the amount in one portion is negligible. This method of cooking is perfectly all right from the point of view of carbohydrate content.

Q: *Besides fruit, what other foods are useful for treats?*
A: Popcorn is one of my child's favorites. Use a low-fat spread rather than butter if you are trying to lower the fat content, or sprinkle with grated cheese or herbs. Other popular snacks are

pretzels, nuts, potato and corn chips, vanilla ice cream (sprinkle diabetic chocolate over it to make it special), waffles topped with ice milk or sugarless pancake syrup, cheese straws made with whole-grain flour, homemade cookies, and diet soda. You can jazz things up to make them more visually appealing. For example, anything with a straw tastes better than the same drink without a straw. A slice of fruit on top of a simple dessert makes it fancy. Ice cubes have great charisma. An ice cube with a sprig of mint or a cherry frozen in the middle decorates a glass of simple fruit punch and makes it special. Be inventive. There is no end to this kind of creativity. If you think about it positively, your child need never feel deprived of the normal pleasures of childhood eating.

Q: *Can you tell me what kinds of low-sugar and low-fat foods are stocked in an ordinary supermarket?*

A: Americans are the luckiest people on earth in this regard. Europeans with diabetes are amazed by the wonderful array of American food products, all neatly labeled with the sugar and fat contents clearly displayed. I strolled around a supermarket in Florida recently and found dozens of fat-, sugar-, and sodium-reduced products. Among these were low-fat spreads made from buttermilk and oil, 2 percent and 4 percent milk, skim-milk cheeses, reduced-fat and -sodium bacon and sausages, low-fat mayonnaise, diet salad dressings, frozen diet dinners, fruits canned in water, sugarless gelatin and pudding desserts, Weight Watchers and similar products, and sugarless jellies and jams. Besides these foods, you have the entire range of fresh fruits and vegetables, whole-grain breads and cereals, lean meats, fish, poultry, cottage cheese, etc., that are naturally low in sugar and fat and high in food value.

Q: *Sometimes the information on the label is confusing. What's the difference between sugar-free and no added sugar, between low-calorie and reduced-calorie, and between sodium-free and low-sodium?*

A: "No added sugar" means that no extra sucrose is added; the product still may have fructose or sorbitol. "Sugar-free" foods are also in this category, so beware. Foods labeled "low calorie" have 40 or fewer calories per serving. "Reduced calories" means that the product has one-third fewer calories than the regular variety. Items labeled "sodium-free" contain less than 5 mg per serving; "very low sodium" means less than 35 mg per serving. "Low sodium" products have less than 140 mg.

Q: *What's the difference between soluble and nonsoluble fiber?*
A: Soluble fiber gets gummy and sticky when cooked. Beans, barley, oatmeal, lentils, and dried peas spring to mind. This type of fiber is extremely nutritious and is helpful in lowering blood glucose and cholesterol. Scientists believe that it can assist in preventing heart disease. Generous and frequent servings of soluble fiber should be incorporated into your family's food plan.

Insoluble fiber is that part of the food that is not digested, but passes out of the body in the stools. This fiber, although not nutritious to humans, plays an important part in the diet because it hastens the passage of other nutrients through the digestive system, thereby protecting against constipation and other disorders.

5

School, Camp, and Exercise

Q: *Should I tell my child's teacher that he has developed diabetes?*

A: You should tell the teacher, the principal, the school nurse, the gym teacher or coach if appropriate, and anyone else who might be involved with your child's health. If possible, ask the principal to set up a meeting for you with those members of the school staff. In fact, not telling the school is grossly unfair to everyone, not the least to your child. There might be a rule against eating in class that he might need to disobey. The candy or glucose tablet in his pocket might be confiscated unwittingly, and a reaction might result. There are also legal problems that might possibly arise. If you should be involved in litigation with the school for any reason, it might be pertinent that they had been informed of the child's condition. The diabetes organizations have pamphlets specifically written to give information to teachers and school staff. You can get these pamphlets by contacting the affiliate nearest you or writing to the Juvenile Diabetes Foundation or the American Diabetes Association main offices. This literature gives much information in an accessible form and is useful for the school to have on file should any questions arise about the care of children with diabetes.

Another person who needs to know that your child has developed diabetes is the school-bus driver. If the child should become ill on the school bus, the driver will need to know what to do. Give the bus driver a sweet drink like Gatorade or a small can of fruit juice or nondiabetic soda to keep for emergencies. If the bus breaks down and has to wait for repairs, the driver should be aware that this might cause a problem for your child. He should know enough about diabetes to make certain that the child is all right and to advise him to eat a snack. Your child, of course, should always have food in his schoolbag or briefcase for unforeseen events.

Q: *Should I give my child's teacher Gatorade or a similar drink to keep in the classroom?*
A: Yes, that's a good idea. The sugar in Gatorade, regular soft drinks, and orange or pineapple juice is rapidly absorbed. There are many one-portion drinks on the market today. Many of these are packed with a straw attached, which makes them very handy. They are useful for the teacher's desk and for the child's bedside table. A quick-witted teacher can head off a situation that could be embarrassing for the child by suggesting that he have a drink. It is difficult for a child to return to class the next day after he has been making a spectacle of himself, perhaps causing the other children to laugh at him. Such a situation only reinforces the idea that he is different, that he cannot function away from Mommy and Daddy, that life is dangerous away from home.

Q: *If my child has an accident at school, will this be more of a problem now that he has developd diabetes?*
A: If he has a small accident—if he cuts or bruises himself, for example—he should be treated by the school nurse in the usual way. Since high blood glucose inhibits healing, it is important that such an accident not be ignored. Cuts and abrasions should be cleaned with antiseptic and covered with a protective bandage. The development of sudden illness, especially vomiting or fever,

should be attended to at once. Protracted vomiting is dangerous for him. Parents should be contacted and every effort made to send the child home. The school office should have the name and telephone number of the child's doctor on file and, in case of emergency, should telephone for instructions.

Q: *Is it safe for my child to participate in strenuous sports at school?*
A: There is no need for the child with diabetes to refrain from any of the usual school sports. On the contrary, exercise is an important part of the control of the condition. A few precautions are necessary, however. He should take extra carbohydrates before strenuous exercise and more afterward. If he is swimming hard, a piece of candy before he enters the pool and an apple or a sandwich when he gets out will keep his blood glucose from dropping below normal. (Just fooling around in the pool, splashing and ducking with friends, or paddling up and down leisurely is not hard work. Extra carbohydrates are needed only for sustained effort.) Don't omit the carbohydrate snack after the exercise is completed. There is often a delayed action for hypoglycemia at this time. Taking extra complex carbohydrates afterward will keep the sugar levels normal.

Q: *What about competitive sports? Suppose he wants to be a member of a sports team that competes against other schools. This can be extremely strenuous and may take place away from home.*
A: Your child must learn to live with his diabetes. It's his for life. If his athletic ability is such that he is chosen to represent his school, this is an important achievement for him. It would be wrong and foolish to discourage him from taking the place that he has earned. He would feel a failure and an invalid. This is exactly what you want to avoid. Let him go, of course, but make sure that a few basic rules are followed.

1. He must bring enough food with him to cover all meals and snacks at their usual hours. (This is something that all the children will be doing anyway. The bus is alive with the crunch of potato chips on these occasions.)

2. He must take extra carbohydrates for the game both before and after.

3. He must tell the coach and one other person about his diabetes. This other person could be his friend.

The friend can be invaluable to the child with diabetes. When his blood-glucose levels fall below normal, the person with diabetes usually becomes fractious. He may not be aware that he needs food. He has to be reminded. The teacher or coach is sitting elsewhere in the bus. He or she is unlikely to know what is happening. The friend sitting beside him is the ideal person to suggest that he eat his snack. I have heard my child's best friend say many a time, "You'd better eat something. You're horribly cross." The teacher or coach will be glad to rely on the observations of the friend. With a bit of help from these two, your child can safely take his place on the team. There are many athletes, even Olympic competitors, who have diabetes.

Q: *Why is exercise important to the diabetic regime?*

A: Large amounts of glucose are required to provide the fuel for vigorous movements. If this glucose were not required by activity, it would accumulate in the bloodstream, where it would cause trouble. Exercise uses up the excess glucose. A person with diabetes who takes regular exercise will find it invaluable in keeping glucose levels normal or close to normal. Children enjoy vigorous activity, and the child with diabetes should be encouraged to partake every day.

Q: *In the winter, it is almost dark when my child returns from school. With homework and television, there is little time for sports. What, if anything, can be done about this?*

A: Perhaps biking to and from school is the answer. Maybe he could walk farther to get the school bus, or, if he is driven to school, be left farther from the building so that he can walk or jog.

If none of these ideas is suitable, how about introducing some sort of family workout at home every day? There are many tapes and videos of aerobics, yoga, and other exercise programs. Don't treat this as part of his diabetes therapy. Introduce it as fun for the family and healthy for father's coronary arteries and mother's desire to fit into her bikini.

Q: *Is there any sort of exercise that is not suitable for him?*
A: Scuba diving and motor racing are better left alone. Skydiving and similar sports should be avoided as well. In these activities, an insulin reaction might be fatal. Swimming alone is unwise for anyone and is discouraged by the Red Cross and other organizations. For a person with diabetes, it is positively dangerous. He should always have a companion and have easy access to sugar should he feel his sugar levels falling. But with proper precautions, swimming is excellent exercise and should be encouraged.

Q: *How can anyone have easy access to sugar while swimming?*
A: Perhaps a small leakproof plastic box could hold a few glucose tablets or candies. This could be left at the side of the pool or even tucked into the bathing suit should the situation demand it, but eating a small bar of chocolate before a long swim is easy enough to do and generally will suffice.

Q: *What about extremely energetic and rough sports like football?*
A: Exercise is such an important part of good diabetes control that any reasonable sport should be encouraged. If your child enjoys playing football, he should be allowed to play football. Since it is so strenuous, it will be necessary to take a few simple precautions, but extra carbohydrates before and after a game is usually sufficient. Diabetes is not a bar to athletic achievement.

Q: *What about activities like Outward Bound that involve danger and self-reliance?*
A: Find out all the details. If your child will be accompanied by

another person, if food and drink can be carried, it is probably all right. Before sending your child off to an Outward Bound program, however, inquire about similar programs for children and teenagers run by the local diabetes organizations. There your child can participate in the same type of activities in safety. This might be a good idea for the first year. Once he has taken part in such a program, he will be better able to handle one for everyone. However, I do not think that activities that require a solo effort in remote places are suitable for a person with diabetes no matter what his age. He needs to be accompanied in case his blood glucose drops below normal. In that situation, perhaps also cold and wet, his mental capacities will be affected temporarily and he may not be able to take the necessary steps to bring his glucose levels up to normal. He needs a companion who will recognize the signs of hypoglycemia and insist that he eat or drink something.

Q: *Can my child go to camp?*
A: The same general attitude can be applied to summer camps. If your child is newly diagnosed, the best thing you can do to help him is to send him to a diabetes camp for the first summer. There he can enjoy all the usual camp activities without worrying. He will also learn about his diabetes and will undoubtedly return home a happier and a healthier child. However, if he has been going to a particular camp for a long time, if he has friends there that he will miss, if his brothers and sisters are going, diabetes should not keep him from attending as well. The camp staff must be made aware, like the school staff, that problems could possibly arise, especially with nighttime hypoglycemia. They must be taught how to cope with it and the child must be allowed to keep food and drink at his bedside, even if this is usually against the rules.

My child attended a diabetes camp in the first year after she was diagnosed at the age of eight. After that, she went to an ordinary camp with her friends. In the four years that she was a camper, she had one bad nighttime reaction after she had refused to eat a meal she didn't like. Her good friend, who slept beside her and was alert to possible problems, woke the counselor. They were unable to persuade her to take some sugar and so phoned a local doctor. (I had provided them with a name and telephone number and had written to the physician in advance.) By the time he arrived, she had fallen asleep and her blood glucose had risen naturally (the body was able to draw on reserves of sugar stored in the liver). When she awoke, she had a headache but little recollection of what had happened. She was able to eat normally, and by afternoon had fully recovered. The camp staff were somewhat upset by the incident but accepted her as a camper for the following year. She had no more problems and looks back on her camp days as a high point of childhood.

Q: *How can I find out about diabetes camps and Outward Bound programs for youngsters with diabetes?*
A: Write to: Camp Directory, National Service Center, American Diabetes Association, 1660 Duke Street, Alexandria, VA 22314.

Q: *Are there any special problems about schools and ordinary camps?*
A: One aspect of diabetes that both the school and camp must know is that the person with diabetes can never miss a meal. The teacher must understand that deprivation of food cannot be tolerated by anyone with insulin-dependent diabetes, and this must never be used as a punishment. He must be allowed to dip into his schoolbag for snacks, even if this is not usually allowed in class. Accordingly, he must be allowed to take food into an examination room, even if taking public examinations such as college boards. If the school has more than one period for lunch, he must be consulted as to which mealtime will suit him best. If his lunch must be a late one, he must be allowed to eat something extra in his classroom. In camp, if a long hike is on the schedule, provision must be made for him to eat at frequent intervals.

Another problem that can arise, especially with the young child, is that the teacher, anxious to help, makes a fuss over the child, insists that he sit in the front of the class, asks him several times a day how he feels, and hovers anxiously like a hen with one chick.

The child feels uncomfortable under such close scrutiny, and his position as "teacher's pet" does not make him popular with his classmates. The child with diabetes has problems enough trying not to feel "different." An overprotective teacher (or counselor, grandparent, aunt, or older brother or sister) can only make things worse. On the other hand, diabetes in the classroom is an excellent opportunity for the teacher to explain the idea of metabolism to the children. A blood-glucose meter is fascinating to school-age children, and they will all want to measure their blood sugar. Many interesting projects for the science table can evolve from learning about little Johnny's diabetes. Taking an interested but matter-of-fact attitude will help the children to accept Johnny's problem and be quick to spot a possible hypo without making the child self-conscious.

Also, the teacher who knows something about diabetes will be on the alert for signs of high blood sugars. The child with diabetes who is suddenly tired, thirsty, asking to go to the bathroom frequently, or who complains of a stomachache is probably suffering from hyperglycemia, or high blood glucose.

Q: *Is he likely to become ill at school?*

A: No. It is rare for a child with diabetes to become ill at school. The most common reasons would be a missed snack, extra exercise, or not eating all his lunch. However, if he should become hypoglycemic in class and have to be sent to the office or the nurse for any reason (perhaps to get some sugar), he must not be sent alone. Another child or a teacher must accompany him. The child whose blood glucose is sinking will become confused easily, and he might not find his way. For the same reason, he must never be sent home during or immediately after an insulin reaction. If he must go home right after the incident, he should be accompanied, preferably by an adult.

Q: *Should the school-age child with diabetes wear an ID bracelet or pendant?*

A: This question is a difficult one. Ideally, yes. All persons with diabetes, especially an older child traveling on public transportation or walking or biking alone, are better protected by an ID bracelet or pendant. In practice, however, it doesn't always work out that way. After my child "lost" three pendants and a half-dozen cards, I finally realized that she resented carrying or wearing one. Children are extremely sensitive about anything that sets them apart.

I think that your child ought to be consulted if he is old enough to have an opinion in this matter. It may be that a young child will be indifferent or will like wearing it. Some older children might like it too. If your child is resistant, however, I wouldn't persist in this. If you encounter hostility to the idea of a piece of jewelry (how about suggesting a long chain to decrease visibility?), perhaps an ID card in the pocket, especially in the pocket of sports clothes, might be acceptable. My daughter agreed after a few years to tuck an ID card into the inside band of her riding hat when she began to ride her pony in jumping competitions.

Q: *Where are identifying cards and jewelry obtained?*
A: If your child attends a special clinic, the diabetes educator or nurse probably has cards. Most of the insulin companies print them to give away. Pendants and necklaces are advertised in the diabetes magazines. They usually are engraved with your child's medical condition. In addition, when you order such a piece of jewelry, one company offers a wallet-size ID card containing a microfilm with information useful in times of emergency such as medical history, insurance, various authorizations, and other essential facts. This would be useful for anyone. Other companies might have other incentives. Check the advertisements in diabetes magazines for the best offers.

Q: *I have been told that stress should be avoided by people with diabetes. Should my child be discouraged from attempting difficult courses so as to reduce the amount of stress on him?*
A: Your child has diabetes, true, but he is still a person, potential worker, spouse, and parent. Education is as important to him as

to anyone else. Diabetes should not be an inhibiting factor in his academic achievement. A recent study of school-age children in England (where public examinations make school life extremely stressful at times) has shown no difference in levels of achievement between children with diabetes and those without. Your child should be discouraged from using his diabetes as an excuse for poor school performance. In fact, if he realizes that he can manipulate the teacher (and children are very quick to realize their advantages) with his diabetes, using it as an excuse for being late, for missing tests or not completing homework assignments, etc., he will turn his attention to you as well. Parents can be manipulated by children very easily. A parent who is already feeling guilty (and which of us is free from guilt as regards our children?) because the child has developed this condition is even more vulnerable. This situation is bad for everyone, but the results are especially destructive for the child. He is not an invalid if you don't make him one, and his diabetes will not affect his ability to cope with normal stress.

Q: *Is boarding school advisable for the child with diabetes?*
A: If the reasons for which the child is boarding are unconnected with his diabetes, I think that the problems of boarding can be overcome with a bit of planning. In the boarding situation, like the camp, the staff have to be fully aware of any possible problems. Whoever is in charge of the dormitory or bedrooms at night must be told that a nighttime insulin reaction might occur and know what to do about it. The child must be allowed to keep food and drink at his bedside, even if this is usually against the rules. The school must be prepared for the occasional unpleasant, even frightening incident of nighttime hypoglycemia and understand that the unreasonable behavior that accompanies these episodes is not to be held against the child.

The school food must be examined carefully. Is it suitable? Very often, school food is disliked by children. The child may eat less than he needs, and a reaction may follow. The child who is boarding must be responsible enough to understand that he must finish his dinner even if he dislikes the food or else must ask for and receive a substitute. It is unreasonable for anyone to expect that the school cook will prepare a different meal to suit one child, but perhaps it can be arranged that a simple dinner (perhaps a frozen one kept in readiness) will be forthcoming in that situation. If it is usual that all the children in the family attend boarding schools, then an effort should be made to control the diabetes in the boarding situation.

One way in which the problems of boarding at school and at camp can be minimized is by use of the pen injector. Since the pen uses only Regular insulin, even though a daily shot of long-acting is given as well, the problem of buildup of insulin in the body overnight is much less. There are fewer nighttime insulin reactions. Also, people using the pen injector are generally testing their blood several times a day, and a low blood glucose at bedtime can be picked up and remedied before it gets out of hand.

It is very important that diabetes should not be seen as a factor that will change everyone's way of life. It is disruptive enough without without making everything else in the family's life subordinate to it. No one benefits from that kind of attention, least of all the child. On the other hand, if boarding school is being considered for the child *because* he has developed diabetes and the parents fear that they cannot cope with the situation, the remedy is much too drastic. The child will resent being sent away because he has presented his parents with a problem that they cannot solve. He has a right to expect that his parents will be able to look after his diabetes at home. A family considering boarding school for this reason needs professional help, and no time should be lost in seeking it.

6

Emotional Problems

Q: *Our family has been turned upside down by diabetes. Is this normal?*

A: I have heard it said that diabetes explodes in a family like a bomb. However, it also carries with it the means of its own repair. Your family will return to normal. Unless we are extremely neurotic, we are all capable of dealing with this problem. Some of us need more help than others, though.

Q: *Do you recommend therapy for the family when a child develops diabetes?*

A: Before considering therapy, I would join a self-help group such as an affiliate of the national diabetes organizations. Most parents find enormous relief from anxiety in the companionship of other people with the same problems. In the group you will find practical help with meal plans and shots, and you will find people who understand your anxieties and will have constructive suggestions to assist you. It is also beneficial to be able to offer advice and assistance to someone else. Your own problems are always reduced when you can help solve someone else's. It is a wonderful psychological mechanism, and I have never known it to fail.

Q: *Suppose that even after joining such a group, parents feel that everyone else is coping but they aren't, that they are in a situation that is beyond their control. What should they do?*
A: It might be a good idea to consider therapy. I would ask advice from the doctor and diabetes educator first, though. The best therapy does not necessarily come from counseling sessions. Sometimes friends and other family members can help. Discuss it between yourselves in the beginning. The child's relationship to his parents and siblings is the key factor.

Q: *My child is angry with me. I feel that he blames me for his diabetes, and I feel guilty. Is this neurotic?*
A: All children blame their parents when things go wrong. This is quite natural. The child sees the parent as invincible. It is a shock to the small child to realize that he has a problem that his mommy and daddy cannot solve. The parents must be prepared for anger, fear, and disappointment. If they are, they can help the child to express them and to get past them. Once past these destructive feelings, the child will be able to comply with the diabetic regime and be fit to control his condition capably.

Q: *How can I help him to express his feelings?*
A: Suggest to him that he is upset and that it is all right to feel that way. Say things like "You must be angry at developing diabetes." . . . "You probably miss eating candy." Bring resentment out into the open and deal with it. Don't hide it. It is not shameful. Avoidance of conflict does not make it disappear; it merely drives it underground, where it will fester and do damage.

Q: *What positive steps can I take to help him to cope?*
A: Expect him to manage his own problems by asking him, "What will you eat at Jimmy's birthday party?" . . . "Will you need extra cookies for school today because you're going swimming?" Doing these things will give him the idea that he is the one who has to work it out. He'll probably come up with a sensible solution and stick to it, because it will be his idea, not yours.

Q: *What about the very young child?*
A: Encourage even the young child to play the dominant role, to be the one who injects rather than the one who is injected. If he is small, give him a syringe (needle removed, of course) to squirt water in the bath, let him treat stuffed toys for diabetes, set up a hospital ward in his playroom. If he is interested, make him a white coat, get him a toy stethoscope. Let him act out the things that frighten him. Overprotection makes things more scary, not less so. It tells the child that Mommy, too, is scared, so the problem must really be terrifying.

Q: *How will this activity help?*
A: It will give him an active rather than a passive role to play. Then continue to emphasize his participation in his diabetic control by encouraging him to do as much for himself as he is able. Even a young child can get out his diabetic kit, wash his hands for his finger prick, swab his injection site with alcohol, be told what his blood glucose is, and be shown how it is entered in his little diary or programmed into his meter. He should be taken to diabetes meetings suitable for his age (there is always the Christmas or Chanukah party of your local affiliate) and allowed to go to the diabetes camp when he is old enough.

Q: *If these things are difficult for a parent to do, does that parent have a problem?*
A: Possibly. Sometimes parents cannot help a child to cope with his fears about diabetes because their own emotional needs intrude. The need of the parent to keep the child helpless, to control him, to use his illness to punish herself or her spouse or to keep the marriage intact will keep her from helping the child to work out his problems. If you think that this might be your situation, then it might be a good idea to consult someone you trust, perhaps a psychologist or a therapist.

Q: *How does having a child with diabetes keep the marriage intact?*
A: It doesn't, but a parent in emotional distress might think it did.

Sometimes a child's illness keeps antagonisms in the marriage from coming to the surface. It is more difficult for a disaffected partner to show anger if his spouse can arouse guilt over the child's condition. Parents in this situation need the child to be helpless, so they resist his attempts at independence. It is not normal to enjoy having an ill child. It is not your life's work. All children grow up and leave home, and any response other than "goody, goody" is suspect. Children with diabetes need extra care and attention, true, but if you find yourself substituting child care for conjugal care, then you should consider getting professional help.

Q: *Does the diabetes itself encourage a neurotic response?*
A: It can. Some people become test-strip junkies. They get things out of proportion, test dozens of times a day, weigh and consider every morsel of food, time their shots to the minute, and refuse to get into any situation that is not in keeping with perfect diabetes control. These people have let diabetes control them instead of controlling the diabetes. Their lives have become dedicated to illness. This does not make for much joy. Parents should keep this situation in mind especially when their children reach adolescence.

Q: *Why are adolescents more vulnerable to the problem?*
A: Adolescence is a difficult time, often characterized by great swings in mood. The teenager is elated one minute, bouncing around on top of the world, and half an hour later, plunged into the depths of despair by some seemingly trivial incident or remark. In the teenager with diabetes, this normal pattern is even more marked because variations in the blood glucose cause mood swings as well. If the adolescent becomes preoccupied with his diabetes, his depression and elation can get out of hand and make him exceedingly unhappy.

Q: *What can parents do to prevent this?*
A: Try to keep a sense of balance and a sense of humor. Al-

though you want your child to look after himself well, you don't want to create a situation where he thinks about nothing but his diabetes. He still has to compete in the real world. He has to do as well as he can in school. He has to develop easy social skills, make friends, get on with people. He has to train for a career, think about marriage and a family, do all the things that other youngsters are doing. Controlling his diabetes should be a skill that he cultivates, but it shouldn't dominate all his thinking. He must learn to work his diabetes control into his ordinary life, not mold his ordinary life around his diabetes control. There is a fine line to be walked here, and the goal of the parent must be to help the child to find that line and to walk on it as comfortably as possible.

Q: *Can the emotional problems of the child with diabetes endanger his life?*
A: They can. Sometimes life is so difficult and unhappy at home that the child manipulates his insulin so that he becomes ill and can escape to the hospital, where he is looked after. In a situation like this, it isn't difficult to misjudge the insulin dose and administer a lethal injection.

Q: *How can parents know if a child is feeling so desperate that he might do such a thing?*
A: Suspect a serious problem if your child has repeated episodes of ketoacidosis. He may be skipping his shot or not eating when he is away from home. Is his lunch money being taken, perhaps by friends on drugs? Has something happened to his insulin supply or his syringes? Perhaps he is afraid that his parents will be angry if he has lost or had his equipment stolen. He may be aware of how expensive it is and feel guilty. Keep your child under close observation if he appears to be unhappy for a long time. Try to win his confidence and get him to tell you what is upsetting him. Perhaps he or she is being hassled at school, teased because of the diabetes, pressured by friends who take recreational drugs, worried about appearance, sexual feelings, poor grades, disease, pregnancy. Whatever is the problem, it is up to

the parent to create an atmosphere where the child can gather the courage to ask for help.

Q: *Is it usual for the diabetes to affect other members of the family such as the brothers and sisters of the child with the condition?*

A: Diabetes in the family affects everyone. Sometimes parents are so anxious about the child with diabetes that the healthy children are neglected. I know a family with two children with diabetes who were happy and well cared for while their healthy sister became delinquent. Unwilling to display hostility toward her siblings, she injured herself, abused drugs, turned to theft, and then became pregnant.

It will not help the child with diabetes if he is pampered and spoiled, if he gets more than he needs of parental attention, especially at the expense of his brothers and sisters. Adult life is difficult for people with diabetes under the best of circumstances, and he needs to be strong and confident to be successful. Overindulgence in childhood will sap his ability to solve problems in later life.

7

Diabetes in the Very Young

Q: *How can diabetes control be measured in the very young child?*
A: Urine can be tested for glucose by squeezing a wet diaper so that the moisture falls onto a testing strip. Disposable diapers are best for this purpose, as there is no danger of soap or detergents affecting the chemistry of the urine. But be sure to remove the layer of treated paper closest to the child's body. This is the film that stays dry even when the rest of the diaper is soaking wet. Discard this and squeeze the rest.

Q: *How often does this have to be done?*
A: Since this procedure is simple, quick, and does not inconvenience the child, I would do it several times a day, noting the times and results in a notebook, which can be kept in the bathroom. A pair of rubber gloves could be kept handy if desired. The frequent tests will give a good indication of the child's glucose levels. Since babies and young children are fed on a fairly regular schedule, the test results will be a reliable guide to adjusting the insulin dose.

Q: *Is urine testing as accurate as blood testing?*
A: Since glucose doesn't spill over into the urine until the blood

levels are twice normal, urine testing cannot tell you that the amount of glucose in the child's blood is too low. Only a blood test can do this. What it *can* tell you is that there is more glucose than the body requires and that you need to take steps to reduce it. Often, the first sign of a feverish illness in the young child is the elevation of the glucose levels and the production of ketones. Frequent urine tests will detect the presence of ketones, which is an indication of trouble.

Q: *Why do ketones indicate trouble?*
A: If ketones are present in the urine, there is not enough insulin in the bloodstream to cope with the glucose. Since extra glucose if often released into the bloodstream during illness, the child may need extra insulin at that time. If you relied on blood testing alone for diabetic control, you might not pick up the presence of ketones.

Q: *How often should urine be tested for ketones?*
A: In the newly diagnosed baby or toddler, your doctor will probably suggest testing often, perhaps several times a day. It is likely that the child had large amounts of ketones at the time of diagnosis. In fact, it was the presence of ketones that gave rise to the symptoms of diabetes: loss of weight, thirst, and fatigue. Once the child's condition is stabilized (usually a matter of a few days), a weekly check will probably suffice. In case of illness, however, ketone levels should be measured several times a day. This will help you to care for the child with a cold or other infection, because it will be a guide to the amount of insulin that is required. Extra insulin is almost always needed during periods of illness, even the most minor.

Q: *Is testing a baby for ketones done in the same way as testing an older child?*
A: You can test for ketones in the same way that you test for glucose. You squeeze a small amount of urine from the diaper onto a small plastic strip that is designed for this purpose. The tip

of the strip is coated with chemicals that will change color if there are ketones present in the urine. Every bottle of strips comes with clear directions. There are strips that test for glucose, strips that test for ketones, strips that test for other problems such as blood or albumin. There are also strips available that are multipurpose. These strips can be "read" for ketones after 15 seconds and glucose after 30 seconds. They are apt to be confusing in the beginning, though. I would suggest that you start out with two separate bottles of strips, one for glucose and one for ketones. When you become more expert at testing, you can use the multifunction strips if you like.

Q: *Can home blood testing be used with young children?*
A: It can. Many doctors recommend taking the drop of blood from the earlobe rather than from fingers. The drop can be extracted more easily if the earlobe or finger is gently warmed before being pricked. A washcloth dipped in warm (not hot) water and wrung out dry can be held on the earlobe to warm it. The baby can be tested after he comes in from outside and his hat is removed. If you are using a finger, it can be immersed in a glass of warm (never hot) water for a minute or two. Make a game of it. Drop a toy into a bowl of water and let him push it around. The blood will come to the surface quickly when the finger is warm.

Q: *How often should the blood of a young child be tested?*
A: It is difficult to make a rule about this. Be guided by the use you can make of the information. A high glucose reading would indicate that more insulin is required; a low reading that less is needed. If you can change the dose and get the expected results from blood testing, then blood testing every day is a good tool for you. However, it doesn't always work out that way with the young child.

Q: *Why not?*
A: The parent has no guarantee that an infant or toddler will eat his full complement of carbohydrates at the next meal. If the

insulin is increased and the child refuses to eat, the parent worries. She knows that he must finish his meal or he will have too much insulin in circulation with insufficient carbohydrates. An insulin reaction may be the result. She may become frantic, trying to get him to finish his bottle or eat a bit more of his solid food. If he refuses, she may try to get him to take his sugar in some other form—juice, candy, soda, etc.—all of which may increase his blood glucose. In the end, she may be no further along than if she hadn't increased his insulin at all. This is much more likely to happen with blood testing, which can fine-tune control, than it is with urine testing, which is a cruder measure. Let common sense be your guide in this as in all aspects of child-rearing. If your child is a good eater, if you can be certain that his appetite on the day in question is normal, testing his blood and adjusting his insulin accordingly will improve diabetes control. However, if his appetite is variable, if he is picky or out of sorts in any way, varying his insulin dose according to the results of frequent blood tests will probably not improve control and might possibly give you an extra problem. You would probably be better off relying on the results of urine tests until he is older.

Q: *Should blood tests be used at all with this age group?*
A: Blood tests are extremely useful in infants to distinguish between periods of crying or crankiness that are due to an imminent insulin reaction from those due to other causes. If a baby is unusually cross, and a check of the blood glucose indicates that glucose levels are abnormally low, giving sugar immediately will avoid an insulin reaction. Since hypoglycemia is a parent's greatest fear in the early years, home blood testing can bring peace of mind.

Q: *Is the equipment expensive?*
A: Not necessarily. Although many parents prefer to have a meter, it is possible to monitor the blood glucose accurately with plastic strips read by eye alone. These strips are reasonably priced. The Sugar-Free Center and other druggists offer discounts on testing strips (see addresses in Appendix 6). Some health-

insurance policies cover most of the cost of blood-testing equipment, including meters.

Q: *Is caring for the infant with diabetes or toddler very difficult?*
A: Because diabetes is unusual in very young children, often the diagnosis isn't made until the child has become quite ill, usually dehydrated. He will have been on an IV in the hospital. After discharge, he may still be thin and debilitated. Often, his appetite is poor. He may be cranky. Injections and blood tests will irk him further. Looking after him will be difficult until he has recovered health and spirits. Parents will worry about whether he is eating enough. The diet sheet provided by the hospital is a good guide. Frequent tests are another. If the family can possibly afford household help, this is the time to get it, even if it is just a teenage girl who comes in after school to play with the child or take him out. Caring for a young child with diabetes is exhausting. Enlist all the friends and relatives you can muster to give you a hand if paid help is impossible.

Q: *How can such a child be persuaded to eat all the carbohydrates that he needs if his appetite is poor?*
A: Small meals offered frequently go down better than larger ones at longer intervals. Give a snack before nap time, too. Make the food look as attractive as possible to tempt him. Finger food might be more appealing to a little child than a formal presentation on a plate. Bananas, plain cookies, milk blended with an egg, orange, and sugar are useful. Ice cream blended with banana and milk is a tempting drink rich in carbohydrates. The food sections of family magazines are full of useful ideas. It is important to remember that these problems will diminish as your child's health returns. When he feels better, he will become more active and his appetite will pick up. Try not to worry.

Q: *If the child is too young to recognize the warning signals of a reaction, how can they be avoided?*
A: Parents need to be extra observant. If his nap is longer than

usual, be suspicious. (Always give food before a nap.) If he loses color or becomes listless after playing happily for a time, check his blood sugar. If possible, make sure that someone is watching him all the time. The other family members can take this in turn. If there are older children, they might be able to help.

Q: *Is it best to keep him close to home?*
A: Not necessarily. Children who are carted around to suit their parents' convenience usually turn out to be more easygoing and flexible than those who are guarded at home. Whatever you do, though, whether it is staying at home or going out, carry food with you. No one with diabetes should venture out of doors without sugar available to him. Carry candy, fruit, juice, crackers, and cookies in your handbag. Keep extra supplies in the car. If you leave your child in someone else's care, make sure that there is food for him at all times.

Q: *Should he be left with a baby-sitter?*
A: It is important that parents should not feel guilty about wanting to go out alone. It is shortsighted and damaging for parents and children alike to focus unduly on the child with diabetes. It will not help him to grow up and be independent if he is given attention that he doesn't need. A teenager with diabetes which is well controlled can be an excellent baby-sitter. He or she is usually tuned in to possible reactions and can take quick averting action. Such a teenager knows how to fill a syringe and give an injection if necessary, although it is unlikely that parents will be content to leave this task to anyone else. Your doctor might be able to recommend a girl or boy for this job.

Another idea is to make an arrangement with the parents of another child with diabetes and sit for each other. This plan saves money as well. If you join your local diabetes self-help group, you will meet others with similar problems, and in helping someone else, you help yourself. Whatever baby-sitting arrangements you make, you should leave clear instructions for the sitter in an obvious place. The refrigerator door is usually a good location. Be very clear as to mealtimes, bedtime, shots to be given, acceptable foods, warning signs of hypoglycemia, telephone number where you can be reached, person to contact in case you cannot be located, telephone number of your doctor, and nearest hospital emergency room. If possible, fill the syringe and prepare any meals in advance. Skip the blood test. Then go out and relax.

Q: *My family is not yet complete. If I have another child, what are the chances that he, too, will develop diabetes?*
A: In diabetes, genetic predisposition is only part of the picture. Others factors need to be present before diabetes develops. Even with identical twins who have the same genetic patterns, the chances that the second twin will develop diabetes is only 30 percent. With fraternal twins or with other children in the family, naturally the chances are greatly reduced. Ninety percent of people who are genetically predisposed to diabetes never develop it. If your child has diabetes and you are inclined not to have any more children only because of the diabetes, you should consult a genetics counselor. The risk is probably far smaller than you think.

Q: *I am a working mother. Is it necessary for me to give up my job to look after my young diabetic child?*
A: The answer to this question is never simple. It really depends on whether or not you can be confident that the person looking after your child is capable of handling the condition. There is nothing sacred in a mother's blood that makes her the only one able to deal with the problem. A grandmother, father, or babysitter might do as well.

Q: *What about a nursery?*
A: It is unlikely that a nursery that looks after many infants will have the staff to do a good job. You may be lucky, however, and find one that is willing to train someone to cope with your baby. If family finances dictate that your job is essential, if you are a one-parent family, or if your job is part of a career pattern that is

important to you, it may be necessary to find someone who is willing and able to learn about diabetic care. Your doctor or hospital social worker may be able to advise you. They might know a retired nurse or other health professional who is looking for such a job. If so, you will have to make sure that this person is willing to familiarize herself with the sort of treatment that your doctor recommends. There has been a revolution in diabetes care in the last few years. A nurse trained many years ago who has not worked with diabetes recently may not be familiar with new injection techniques, new ideas in diet, testing procedures, and other matters. Your helper must be willing to learn from you. In diabetes, ignorance is never bliss. Fortunately, there are many resources available to you both. In addition to books like this one written for the lay person, there are organizations such as the Juvenile Diabetes Foundation (address in Appendix 6) and the American Diabetes Association that you can join to meet other people who care for children with diabetes. You might suggest that your helper join with you to keep abreast of the latest ideas, techniques, and literature and to meet other people who have similar problems. It is always useful to know others in the same boat. The solutions they have found may be of value to you, and they provide an enormous amount of moral support.

8

The Teen Years

Q: *Is diabetes more difficult in adolescence?*

A: Everything is more difficult in adolescence. It is hard for the teenager to cope with all the strange and exciting things that are happening to his body. It makes him moody and hard to live with. If he has to cope with diabetes as well, it imposes a great strain. I have seen many a cheerful, compliant child who has been keeping to his food plan, testing his blood at home, and presenting a picture of cooperation change almost overnight into a sullen, stubborn adolescent, snapping at his mother, "forgetting" his record book, avoiding the doctor's eye, and refusing to see the dietician. This is all quite normal. There is no need for parents to be embarrassed at the attitude of this newly grown monster. In a few years, he or she will revert to the pleasant, cooperative person who is hiding inside that teenage dragon. The important thing to remember about adolescence is that it is not permanent. Try to keep your sense of humor intact even if your child appears to have lost his.

Q: *Can anything be done to ease the teenager through this period?*

A: One thought that might be helpful to parents of the newly diagnosed child with diabetes is to be sure to let the diabetes be *his,* not yours. If you take over control completely, when it comes time to rebel against your authority, he will rebel against the diabetes as well. No matter how young the child, it is important that he be permitted to handle things as soon as he is able. Even if the parent can do it better or more quickly, so long as he is capable of doing it safely, he should be allowed. It is the role of the parent to teach him to look after himself, not to do everything for him.

Even young children can get their own snacks, keep their diabetic kit in order, and learn the exchange value of everyday foods. A school-age child can become expert. He should be encouraged to learn as much as possible about diabetes. There are many excellent books written for children that can probably be found in your specialist clinic, the local library, or through the diabetes magazines. When he has learned a little, he should be consulted when his regime has to be changed. It is quite in order for parents to say, "You've had two reactions this week. What do you think you could do to prevent any more?" *Diabetes Forecast* has articles and stories for children. They solicit letters and drawings from them as well. There are contests to enter, prizes to win, pen pals to meet. Encourage your child to participate. If you join your local affiliate, he can get pleasure from helping to raise money for diabetic research. Good attitudes developed in childhood will make the teenage years less painful.

Q: *Does sleeping late in the morning on weekends and holidays affect control?*

A: Diabetes is thrown off balance by missed snacks, late meals, and delayed injections. This can be a problem in adolescence, when sleeping late seems to be a necessary pleasure. The best solution is probably a compromise. Allow an extra hour in bed on a weekend morning. If he wants to have more than an extra hour in bed (and who doesn't?), he will have to compromise a little too.

Let him get up, take his shot, fix himself a breakfast tray, and take it back to his room. After he has eaten, he can lounge about in his bedroom, even go back to sleep if he likes, and still not disturb his diabetic control.

Q: *Is control upset during adolescence owing to physical changes in the child?*

A: Yes. Many girls will find that diabetic control becomes erratic during the menstrual period. Extra finger pricks are a good idea on those days so that insulin needs can be ascertained. Stress is a factor in control as well. In periods of stress, the blood glucose rises. Hyperglycemia (high blood glucose; see Appendix 3 for symptoms and treatment) may result. Since the teen years are a stressful time, episodes of hyperglycemia are often more frequent than in childhood. Growth hormones and sex hormones play havoc with control as well. This can usually be coped with by increasing the insulin, although one should be careful not to create a situation in which the adolescent is overinsulinized. This can lead to weight gain.

During adolescence, it is especially important that good relations have developed between the teenager and the doctor so that problems such as overweight can be discussed and dealt with. Often, the physician, satisfied that the teenager (usually a girl) is not statistically overweight according to his chart, dismisses her unhappiness about her shape as nonsense. To the teenage girl, desperate to compete in the popularity stakes at school, this can be the source of much unhappiness and lead to obsessions with diet or even to other problems such as anorexia or bulimia. These conditions, dangerous for anyone, are fatal to the person with diabetes. It is especially important, if your teenager is on intensive therapy of four or more injections a day, to make sure that there is no excessive weight gain. On intensive therapy, hunger and appetite increase because of extra insulin. Since blood-glucose levels are better controlled, less glucose is lost in urine. If your child is on intensive therapy, speak to the doctor about reducing overall calories and increasing exercise. Be careful not to overtreat episodes of hypoglycemia.

Q: *Is this a drawback to intensive therapy?*
A: No. Intensive therapy with pump, pen, or button infuser can bring about excellent control. It is just a point to watch out for.

Q: *Are teenagers with diabetes more subject to moodiness than others?*
A: Adolescence is a time of great mood swings anyway, but diabetes seems to make it worse. If the blood glucose drops during the night, the teenager usually wakes up feeling cranky and short-tempered. Too much insulin makes him hungry and too little makes him tired. Boys worry that diabetes might affect their popularity or athletic ability, and girls worry about gaining too much weight or having a defective baby. It is a difficult time for them, and parents have to be patient and try to see things from their point of view.

Q: *Will diabetes affect the sex life of the young adult?*
A: I don't see any reason why it should.

Q: *What about impotence? I have heard that diabetes can cause impotence in men.*
A: Impotence can be a problem for men with diabetic neuropathy of long standing. I have never heard of a young male becoming impotent. And now, with enormous research going on in the field of diabetic neuropathy, it is likely that this problem will be solved before long.

Q: *Can diabetes affect menstruation?*
A: The onset of menstruation is sometimes delayed in the girl with diabetes. Once menstruation begins, however, there should be no special problems resulting from the diabetes. The possible delay in beginning menstruation should be explained to girls, who

usually look forward eagerly to their first period and spend much time in the preteen years discussing this with their friends. It can be disappointing to a young girl to feel that she is being left behind when all her friends are becoming women. She should be reassured that her time will come even if it is postponed somewhat. In this area, too, good control plays a part.

Q: *Are there other problems associated with growth and sexual development?*
A: It is rare today for diabetes to affect growth, unless control has been exceptionally erratic in the early years. Your child will be weighed and measured at every visit to the diabetic doctor, and his growth will be carefully noted. If you are anxious on this point, discuss it with the doctor. Some parents are so worried about taking up the doctor's time that they feel timid about asking questions that aren't specifically medical. Sometimes the doctor has more patients to see than he can manage in his office hours; he looks rushed and doesn't encourage conversation. If this is the situation in your doctor's office, write down your questions at home when you are relaxed. That way the doctor's attention can be directed to the important issues that worry you without any time-consuming preliminaries. Also, remember that in diabetes, more so than in most medical specialties, the patient's care is shared by the entire team. The nurse, the diabetes educator, the dietician are all involved in looking after your child. It is my experience that these health-care professionals know a great deal about diabetes. Some of them have diabetes themselves, and that is why they have chosen this career. They are especially motivated to help, and anxious parents will find them a great source of comfort.

Q: *Should teenagers with diabetes be sexually active?*
A: In my view, no young teenage girl should be sexually active, because, among other reasons, of the risk of developing cancer of the cervix in later life. But I know that this is almost impossible

to enforce. In sex, even more than in other aspects of life, the pressure of the peer group is dominant. As far as the diabetes is concerned, however, it should not make a difference.

Q: *Can a girl with diabetes take the contraceptive pill?*
A: Most doctors agree that there is no increased risk to diabetics in using the pill, especially the low-dose pill. Other types of birth-control devices, such as the coil, the diaphragm, and condom, however, have a certain advantage in that one can stop using them without having to take the blood glucose into consideration. What should be emphasized to girls is that it is important that glucose levels be normal *before* conception, so *planning* is essential and an early consultation with the doctor before conception is strongly advised. Pregnancy is one area where the pump has proved to be extremely useful.

Q: *Is pregnancy difficult, even dangerous, for girls and women with diabetes?*
A: The management of the diabetic pregnancy has improved enormously in the past few years. Today, specialist prenatal diabetic clinics have demonstrated that on a regime of three or four shots a day, the mother-to-be with diabetes can keep her glucose levels normal during pregnancy.

Q: *Can she have a normal delivery?*
A: More women with diabetes are having normal, vaginal deliveries than ever before. Women with diabetes used to produce large babies, which made cesarean sections almost obligatory. With better control during pregnancy, babies can be kept to normal size.

Q: *What caused babies to be so large?*
A: High maternal blood glucose during pregnancy caused the babies to gain more weight than normal. That is one reason why it is essential to maintain normal glucose levels.

Q: *Why is it important to have normal glucose levels at the time of conception?*
A: It is less likely that the infant will be born with birth defects if glucose levels are normal before conception and maintained that way for the entire pregnancy.

Q: *Is this difficult?*
A: Women are motivated during pregnancy to look after themselves better. Increasing the number of shots and doing several finger pricks a day can usually keep the blood glucose normal. During pregnancy, hormonal changes make diabetes control easier. If normal glucose levels are maintained before and throughout the pregnancy (and they can be), the outcome should be no different than if the woman did not have diabetes.

Q: *Can the mother with diabetes breast-feed her baby?*
A: There is no reason why the mother with diabetes should not breast-feed her baby. She may have to increase the number of calories she eats, and therefore a slight increase in insulin may be necessary too. After delivery, however, frequent changes of insulin are necessary to adjust to the nonpregnant state. Hormonal changes in the first few days after the birth will result in changes in insulin requirements.

Q: *Will the pregnant woman with diabetes have to be admitted to the hospital early?*
A: This is a possibility. The doctor may want to admit her in order to keep things under tight control. Also, if she has had any trace of high blood pressure, this may be necessary. However, some prenatal diabetic clinics allow patients with diabetes to wait for full term at home if there are no problems.

Q: *Will the birth be induced?*
A: When babies of mothers with diabetes were almost always larger than normal, it was the custom to deliver them before full term, sometimes by induction but more usually by cesarean sec-

tion. In some hospitals, this practice is still common, even though there is less need for it. Take time to choose an obstetrician in whom you have confidence and who is willing to discuss the matter with you. Although the doctor will always reserve the right to do whatever seems medically advisable at the time of delivery, an obstetrician should take into consideration the patient's view in the matter. Ask your diabetes doctor to refer you to a specialist diabetes prenatal clinic if there is one in your area. There you will probably find the most up-to-date methods and the most sympathetic service.

Q: *Is there a chance that the baby will develop diabetes?*
A: The chance is small. It should not be a deterrent to having a family. There are many factors involved here. One of them is whether the father or the mother has diabetes. If only the mother has diabetes, the chances of the child's developing diabetes are lower than if the father had the condition. If you are worried about this, ask your diabetes doctor to refer you to a genetics counselor before you embark on a pregnancy.

Q: *Can a woman with diabetes have an abortion?*
A: Women with diabetes can have abortions just like nondiabetics. It is very important, though, that any operation requiring a general anesthetic be performed in a hospital and that the staff be aware that the patient is an insulin-dependent diabetic. Abortion, though, is traumatic for everyone. Even if the pregnancy is legally terminated for medical reasons, it is a situation that is fraught with problems.

Q: *Even if the girl is young, unmarried, and has diabetes?*
A: A girl's best friend should be her mother. If mothers strive to keep open the channels of communication between themselves and their teenage daughters, it is less likely that girls will become pregnant out of ignorance or spite. Sometimes young pregnant girls are secretly pleased by the prospect of thwarting domineering parents or by the thought of having someone who will be

helpless and dependent on them. Adolescence is a time of expansion and experimentation, but it is also a time when the security of childhood is still required. Give your teenager room to try new ideas and independence, but always make sure that the way back to you is left open. The young person with diabetes needs this reassurance even more, because for him or her the road to independence is more precarious.

Q: *Can emotional problems during adolescence interfere with diabetes control?*
A: Yes. A recent study shows that teenage girls who are anxious and depressed (perhaps about grades, popularity, or weight) have higher blood-glucose levels. Boys fare better. This may be because boys tend to get more exercise during adolescence than girls. In fact, aerobic dancing, which has an appeal for girls, can be helpful in promoting exercise among teenage girls.

Q: *Are there other emotional problems associated with diabetes in the teen years?*
A: Teenagers are absorbed with their bodies. This adult body is new to them and infinitely interesting. They spend much time washing it, dressing it, and decorating it with cosmetics. Diabetes has a negative body image. Girls worry that pregnancy will be a problem for them. They may feel less feminine because of this. An insulin reaction can make the teenage boy feel weak and dependent instead of strong and manly. Junk food, so beloved by the adolescent, has to be eaten sparingly. Cigarettes, booze, and drugs, the passport to acceptance in some circles, must be avoided. The adolescent who fears that he or she won't be popular if the diabetes is known will hide it.

Q: *Are there problems at home as well?*
A: Children with diabetes are often both pampered and restricted at home. Other children in the family can resent the time and attention given to them, so sibling sympathy and support, so necessary to the young person, is often lost.

Q: *Would it be better for students with diabetes to attend college near home rather than go far way, where they would be in complete control of their condition without any help?*
A: If your teenager has been taught how to look after himself from the time that he is first diagnosed, he should be quite able to care for himself by the time he reaches college age. The decision about which college or university to attend is a scholastic (and financial), not a medical, decision. It may be that only a particular institution offers the curriculum he wants. He may be looking forward (he *should* be looking forward) to the opportunity to live in a new place, make new friends, and be more independent. His diabetes should not rob him of that chance. If it does, he is likely to rebel against it. Besides, he will not be in complete control of his condition. He will have friends and acquaintances. He will also be able to arrange medical help at the college. You and he, with advice from the doctor, should be able to arrange for him to attend a diabetic doctor or a specialist clinic near the college. He will be able to have copies of his records transferred there. He should also find a friend who is willing to learn about the diabetes and can help him.

Q: *Should he have a roommate?*
A: It is usual for freshmen to share rooms, so you can leave this problem to the college authorities. Certainly, it is a good idea and one that he should continue throughout his school career if he likes it. It is a good way of ensuring that someone will always be aware if he has a problem like a nighttime reaction. However, if he is a solitary type or hasn't found a companion with whom he would like to share a room, he might prefer to ask a neighbor to keep an eye on him. If he is mature enough to live away from home, he must be mature enough to ask for this kind of assistance without embarrassment.

Q: *Is the food suitable in college cafeterias?*
A: It may not be exactly the same as home, but the choice is usually wide enough so that the student with diabetes can stay

within his meal plan. College students tend to drink a lot of coffee and tea, often in late-night study sessions. Excess caffeine can affect insulin absorption, so it would be better for them to use decaffeinated brands.

Q: *Is alcohol a problem for people with diabetes?*
A: Although many people with diabetes drink alcohol, drinking can be a problem. There are many reasons for this. One reason is that alcohol can bring on a reaction. If a person becomes hypoglycemic after drinking, it will appear to others (perhaps the police) that he is drunk and disorderly. His diabetes may not be apparent even if he has an ID card in his pocket or a bracelet around his wrist simply because the arresting officer might never think to look for it. He may be put somewhere to "sleep it off," and he could go into a coma. Tragedy could be the result.

People with diabetes should drink only with food and never instead of food. Drinking on an empty stomach is a prescription for disaster, as it lowers the blood glucose exceedingly fast. Food should be eaten before any alcohol is drunk. The alcohol itself should be counted as a fat exchange. Alcohol raises fat levels, which may contribute to diabetic nerve disease. In this way, it can be related to impotence, which might be an argument for you when convincing your teenager not to go on a binge.

Q: *What about diabetic beer?*
A: Diabetic beer contains less carbohydrates than other beers, just as much alcohol, and just as many calories. It should not be regarded as a safe substitute.

Q: *What drink is the safest?*
A: Spritzers, dry wines, and spirits mixed with sugar-free mixers are probably best. Avoid drinks that are very sweet such as fortified wines like sherry and port, sweet dessert wines, and all whiskey, gin, and vodka mixed with ordinary sodas. My own daughter, now at the age where these activities are important, switches to

mineral water with ice and lemon after the first drink and tells me that no one ever notices. Heavy drinking among the young is less fashionable now than it was a generation ago.

Q: *What advice can you give to a young person wishing to go out with friends to a roadhouse, nightclub, or bar?*

A: **1.** Let your friends know that you have diabetes and exactly what this means regarding alcohol.

2. Eat a good meal before you go out.

3. Drink moderately. One or two beers is enough.

4. Eat something with the drinks. A bag of potato chips would help. Most cocktail bars serve peanuts, pretzels, and olives. Nibble these freely.

5. Don't miss any meals or snacks while you are in the bar.

6. If the drinking session goes on for a long time and you don't want to leave early, switch to a sugar-free soft drink. If the others are drinking gin, whiskey, or rum, no one will notice that yours is only a mixer. If they are drinking cans of beer, sip yours slowly. It is never adult to make yourself ill. It's stupid. Anyway, it's better to pass up on a few drinks than become unpopular because friends must cope with frequent insulin reactions.

Q: *What shall I do if my teenager comes home drunk?*

A: Make sure that he isn't having a reaction. Do a finger prick. If his glucose is normal, let him sleep for a while. If it is low, try to get him to take sugar. Treat it as an insulin reaction.

Q: *Is it dangerous for people with diabetes to abuse drugs?*

A: Yes, very dangerous. The most important elements in good diabetes control are balance and regularity. Drug abuse is a major disturbance to the body. Parents cannot be too emphatic in explaining this to their children. Drug-taking is absolutely incompatible and may even be life-threatening to a person with diabetes.

Q: *Is this true for marijuana as well as the harder drugs?*
A: Yes. Even with a drug that may only induce a mild euphoria, he may forget to eat or take shots. Warning symptoms of an impending reaction may go unnoticed. He may find himself popular in dubious company, such as drug users, because he has access to needles and syringes. There is nothing in the drug scene that could be advantageous to him.

Q: *What should a parent do if there is a suspicion that the teenager with diabetes is experimenting with drugs?*
A: Contact your diabetes doctor and discuss the matter with him or her and the staff. They may have other patients with the same problem. It may be necessary to inform the authorities. Parents cannot cope with this situation by themselves. It requires expert handling.

Q: *How can parents convince a teenager whose friends abuse drugs that he must not indulge?*
A: A teenager is old enough to live with the knowledge that diabetes is a potentially fatal disease. Only careful management on his part is keeping him alive. If he opts out of this management, he will not survive. Drug abuse is opting out. It is my experience that most young people are frightened by drugs and will seize on any excuse to reject them provided that the excuse is acceptable to their friends. Diabetes must be seen as an acceptable excuse. Perhaps a family friend, an older person with diabetes, or the doctor could convince your child that it is okay to say no. At this sensitive age, a teenager may accept advice more easily from someone outside the family. Try to find someone whom he particularly admires and ask that person to talk to him. Perhaps a teacher, social worker, or sympathetic policeman may be the right person to help. This is an especially difficult problem if drug abuse is normal behavior in your neighborhood. If so, you might examine your options. Is it possible for you to move?

Q: *Should someone with diabetes smoke?*
A: No. Diabetes is a risk factor in the development of heart disease. Smoking is also a risk factor. The combination could be significant. Smoking constricts the small blood vessels, decreasing circulation. This applies to pipe, cigar, and cigarette smoking, and to chewing tobacco. It also contributes to stillbirths, miscarriages, premature babies, and babies with birth defects. Fifteen to 20 percent more insulin is needed by diabetics who smoke. This extra insulin can contribute to unwanted weight gain. Because it is so difficult to give up, it should never be started.

Q: *How can I discourage my teenager from smoking when other members of the family smoke?*
A: You can't. Children tend to do what we do rather than what we say. If you want to make sure that your child with diabetes does not smoke (or drink or abuse drugs), you should not do these things yourself.

Q: *Is it all right for teenagers with diabetes to attend discos and parties that go on for long periods and where alcohol is served?*
A: By disco-going age, your child should be ready to take charge of his diabetes himself. It is really up to him to demonstrate that he knows how to cope with late hours, frantic activity, and excitement. Disco dancing uses up a lot of energy and probably requires extra carbohydrates. This would be available in the form of soft drinks and snacks. Excess alcohol can be refused, and an occasional late night will not upset the diabetes control. Denying him permission to do what is normal for his age will upset his control more.

In this situation, as in many others in childhood and adolescence, the child's best friend can be a great help. If the friend can be persuaded to take an interest in diabetes, perhaps be given books to read if that is appropriate or even be invited to accompany your child on various outings sponsored by the diabetes organizations, this can be an advantage. I know one child with diabetes whose best friend can fill the syringe, do finger pricks, count exchanges, and recognize the signs of an impending reaction. With this friend, the child with diabetes has successfully gone on camping trips for a week at a time, hiked long distances, and competed in sports competitions far from home.

Q: *At what age should the teenager with diabetes be allowed to vacation alone away from home?*
A: No matter what the child's age, it is a good idea to let the first period away from home after diagnosis be one in which the diabetes can be looked after by trained medical staff. The diabetes camp is ideal for this purpose. Children up to late teens can be accommodated. Here they can participate in all sorts of social and athletic activities confident that help is at hand if required. The camp gives the newly diagnosed child the opportunity to learn more about his diabetes in an environment in which he is no different from anyone else and where the role models, the successful, glamorous counselors and staff, often have diabetes themselves. This helps most children and teenagers to come to terms with the condition. It also gives parents a much-needed break, especially needed at this time when life is particularly stressful and bewildering.

Q: *Should the teenager with diabetes be allowed to drive a car?*
A: Driving is important in our culture. It is regarded by teenagers as a coming-of-age ceremony, a rite of passage from childhood to adult life. Refusing him permission to drive will only cause him to feel deprived and resentful. I would allow it provided that he can demonstrate, to your complete satisfaction, that he is looking after himself responsibly. He must be willing to do a finger prick before he gets behind the wheel and take appropriate food or drink if his blood glucose is below 72 mg/dl. Low blood glucose will impede his reactions and possibly cause an accident.

Q: *Can he get car insurance?*
A: Yes, but his rates may be higher. Before you buy insurance, check with your local affiliate. They may be able to recommend

a company that gives insurance to drivers with diabetes at reasonable rates.

Q: *Does he have to inform anyone that he has diabetes when applying for a driver's license or insurance?*
A: If there is a question on the form asking this, he must answer it truthfully. If he does not, his insurance will not be valid and, should he have an accident (even one unconnected with the diabetes and in which he is completely blameless), his insurance will be void.

Q: *Will he have to present medical evidence to get his license?*
A: It varies from state to state, naturally, but most require a letter from the doctor saying that the diabetes is under control.

Q: *What about driving a motorcycle?*
A: Much as parents shrink from the thought of this with all its attendant dangers, the same principle prevails. If he would be allowed to do this if he didn't have diabetes, his diabetes should not be allowed to stand in the way. If he is responsible enough to do frequent finger pricks, not drive if his blood glucose is below 72 mg/dl, carry sugar with him at all times and take some at the first sign of a reaction, carry an ID card or wear identifying jewelry, then permission should be given or withheld on the same grounds that it would be if he did not have diabetes.

Q: *Does the diabetes have to be declared to the motor vehicle bureau for a motorcycle license?*
A: If there is a question on the application form about disqualifying diseases, he must declare the diabetes. However, a letter from the doctor will probably satisfy the authorities.

Q: *Are there any jobs barred to people with diabetes?*
A: Yes. A diabetic cannot work as an interstate trucker, fly a commercial airplane, be a steeplejack, or work as a paramedic. He may be accepted into the armed forces, but it would probably be

into a specialized category. It is unlikely that he could be in the police. But the number of jobs that he can do is legion. The medical profession is an excellent choice; doctors, nurses, diabetes educators, dieticians, and researchers all do well. In any job connected with diabetes, having the condition oneself is an added advantage. Exercise physiology, sports medicine, physical therapy, and health administration are good choices as well for anyone interested in careers in medicine. People with diabetes work as farmers, teachers, secretaries, salespersons, artists, lawyers, architects, actors, professional athletes; almost any line of work has people with diabetes in it. Your youngster should never feel that diabetes has seriously limited his choice of career.

9
Traveling

Q: *What would happen if my child with diabetes became ill while traveling overseas?*
A: To avoid problems, it is sensible to obtain a travel card. Send 15 cents and a self-addressed envelope to: Diabetes Alert Card, American Diabetes Association, 1660 Duke Street, Alexandria, VA 22314.

You will receive a special document for your child giving the following message in Bengali, Dutch, Finnish, French, German, Italian, Japanese, Norwegian, Portugese, Serbo-Croatian, Spanish, Swedish, and Urdu:

> I have diabetes and am on daily insulin/oral hypoglycemic agents. If I am found ill, please give me 2 tablespoons of sugar, preferably in water. There should be sugar in my pocket or bag. If I am unconscious or do not recover, please call a doctor or an ambulance.

In addition to this useful card, it is wise to have a letter written by your doctor on official stationery (his or a hospital's) stating that you need to carry syringes, needles, insulin bottles, etc., for your child in your bag. There is always a danger, especially in underdeveloped countries, that these supplies will be mistaken by Customs for drug-abuse equipment. A letter from the doctor translated into the appropriate language is useful, especially when your child is old enough to travel without you.

Q: *Where can I get such a letter?*
A: Your doctor can supply the English text, of course. A travel agent might be able to suggest a translator. Perhaps a foreign student or shopkeeper can help. If you cannot find anyone suitable, contact the nearest college or university where courses are offered in the language you require. As a last resort, you can write to the consulate or embassy of the country you propose to visit. Allow plenty of time for a reply.

Q: *What extra equipment do I need to carry for my child when traveling?*
A: Take plenty of everything. Remember that insulin strengths in Europe (except the United Kingdom and Ireland) are different from those in the United States, Canada, and Australia. If you need to buy extra insulin on the European continent, you will have to by it in 40 or 80 strengths and estimate the proper dosage. You will also have to buy special U40 or U80 syringes. Why give yourself that worry? Anticipate breaking or losing a few bottles and bring plenty of extras. Even if you have a blood-testing meter, you might find it handier to carry the strips you read by eye while traveling. Or take both, just to be sure. Pack all your equipment in two bags, each set complete down to the last detail. Keep one set on your person at all times. If you are traveling with another adult, give that person the second set. That way, you can be certain that missing baggage won't throw you into a panic and spoil your vacation. Naturally, you should not pack insulin in a bag that is destined for the hold of an airplane, because of the dangers of freezing. Keep all insulin bottles in your hand baggage at all times, stored in an insulated traveling case.

Q: *Will going through the x-ray machines at the airport affect the insulin?*
A: No.

Q: *Will it affect a pump?*
A: Check with the manufacturer.

Q: *Will insulin keep in a hot climate?*
A: According to the manufacturers, it will keep stable in temperatures up to 25 degrees Celsius for a month. However, try to keep it as cool as possible without freezing. If there is no refrigerator or icebox available, bring an insulated picnic bag from home or buy an insulated insulin carrier advertised in the diabetes magazines. This is a bag designed especially for holding insulin vials and has pockets for syringes and swabs as well. Make certain that, if your traveling case has sachets of frozen material to keep the bag cool, the insulin bottles never come into contact with those sachets. Freezing destroys insulin. If a bottle should freeze accidentally, discard it. If you have no other means of keeping insulin cool, wrap the bottles in wet cloth. Keep the cloth wet all the time. The constant evaporation of the water will cool the bottle in the same way that panting cools a dog. Don't leave insulin in either the glove compartment or the trunk of the car, as these areas heat up quickly in the sun.

Q: *Can you give me a checklist for traveling?*
A: Twice as much insulin as you think you will need
Glucagon
Extra syringes and needles
Urine-testing strips for glucose and ketones
Blood-testing strips
Finger pricker, lancets, or needles
Alcohol swabs
Injector if needed (an extra if possible)
ID card and letter if traveling abroad

Travel medical insurance
Food and drink in quantity

Q: *Are there any special problems about taking shots in an aircraft?*
A: Because there is less resistance at high altitudes, you need only half as much air injected into the bottle.

Q: *How does one cope with changes of mealtimes while on the plane?*
A: Keep your watch set to home time until you arrive, so that you can be certain that your child is eating on schedule. Do frequent finger pricks while on board the plane and use Regular insulin in small amounts to keep the blood glucose normal.

Q: *What about crossing time zones?*
A: If your child is on a single shot of Regular and NPH/lente per day, do the following:

Going eastward (from California to New York or from America to Europe), you will find that the day is shortened so that the next shot will be due less than twenty-four hours after the last one. To cope with this, take extra carbohydrates with the meal (supplementing from your store of goodies if necessary), in case there is any insulin left over in his bloodstream from the last shot. When you arrive, change your watch to local time and proceed normally, checking the blood glucose often to ensure that there is no problem.

Going westward (from New York to California or from Europe to America) the day will become longer. You will probably have an extra meal. Give the child a few units of extra insulin initially and feed him every three hours to prevent an insulin reaction. Check blood glucose often and keep sugar handy to forestall a problem. If glucose levels are high the next day, add a small amount of extra insulin.

If your child injects twice a day with a mixture of Regular and NPH/lente, do the following:

Going eastward, the day is shorter. Give the normal shot in the morning and reduce the evening shot by 10 percent. For flights longer than twenty-four hours, omit the NPH or lente and use only Regular insulin, giving a small shot before each meal. Test before you inject to get dose right.

Going westward, the day is longer. Give the shots at the usual time. (Your watch is still on home time.) Before the next meal is served, give another shot of Regular insulin.

If your child is on multiple-injection therapy with a pump, pen, or button infuser, consult your doctor before setting off for instructions regarding the adjusting of the long-acting insulin. Give Regular 30 minutes before each meal as usual.

Q: *Is eating in restaurants a problem?*

A: In vacation places that are crowded, plan to eat before or after peak times to avoid delays.

In the Third World, avoid any food that might possibly be contaminated by unhygienic handling or inadequate cooling. Don't eat undercooked meat, shellfish, milk and milk products including cream sauces and whipped cream, soft cheeses, peeled fruits, slices of melon or pineapple, or leafy vegetables. Don't use ice cubes and drink only bottled water, even for brushing your teeth. Bring plenty of snacks from home: cheese, crackers, peanut butter, fruit juices, plain cookies. Eat only fruit that you peel yourself, cooked vegetables, rice, well-cooked meat and fish, bread, and cooked starches like yams or plantains.

Q: *Will traveling to a different climate make the diabetes unstable?*

A: Test frequently. You may have to adjust the insulin dose a little. In hot climates, less insulin is usually required. Since you have plenty of testing strips, however, more frequent finger pricks shouldn't be a problem.

Q: *What other preparations should be made for unforeseen events?*

A: Change some money into the local currency before you set out so that if there are delays leaving the airport or getting to your destination, you can always buy food. Have small coins for the telephone, as well.

Q: *If my child has to have immunizations for travel to less healthful parts of the world, will these upset the diabetes?*
A: Different immunizations have different effects. To avoid any problems that might spoil your vacation, get all immunizations as far in advance of traveling as possible.

Q: *Will strange food upset the diabetes?*
A: Even though the cuisine is different, you'll probably find that the basic foodstuffs are familiar. So long as you can recognize a carbohydrate when you see one, this shouldn't be a problem. And the staple of all countries is carbohydrates, whether it be bread, rice, yams, or pasta.

Q: *If my child should need a doctor when we are abroad, how can we find one who speaks English?*
A: English is the lingua franca for educated people in most parts of the world. But the following organizations may be able to recommend physicians experienced in diabetes:

International Association for Medical Assistance for Travelers
736 Center Street
Lewiston, New York 14092

IDF International Association Center
40 Washington Street
1050 Brussels, Belgium
Tel: 32-2-647-4414

Intermedic
777 Third Avenue
New York, NY 10017
Tel: 212-486-8974

10

Medical Costs, Insurance, Research, and Development

Q: *How much will it cost to look after our child's diabetes?*
A: Naturally, there is a great variation in cost depending on where you live, what kind of insurance you have, and what level of technology you choose to use. Basically, all persons with diabetes have to buy insulin and syringes. They should also, as minimum care, see the doctor every three months, have certain laboratory tests, and buy equipment for blood and urine testing. Certain aids such as alcohol swabs, meters, log books, magazine subscriptions, and camps can be said to be optional, although, if you can afford them, you might find them well worth the money. An ordinary notebook can be used for keeping a log, testing strips can be read by eye, magazines can be borrowed, alcohol and cotton can be used instead of swabs, and it is possible, in some states, to get help with camp fees.

Let's look at what diabetes cost in 1988 for a child of seven living in Massachusetts, taking three shots a day and doing three finger pricks a day (data from Diabetes Forecast).

	(In $)
insulin	98
syringes	216

4 lab tests	68
4 doctor's visits	384
alcohol swabs	24
test strips	528
lancets	132
miscellaneous (batteries, glucagon, and logbooks)	160
total	$1,610

Not included: meter, diabetes education, subscription to magazines, and camp.

Of this $1,610 paid out in 1988, the health-insurance policy covered $1,048, leaving $562 for the family to pay.

Q: *How can costs be reduced?*
A: Since hospital admissions are exceedingly expensive, costs can be reduced by frequent testing to prevent problems. One admission for ketoacidosis can cost $1,000. A meter costs about $200. Strips to be read by eye cost less than 50 cents each. Prevention is always better than cure.

Let your doctor, diabetes educator, or social worker know if you have money worries.

Shop around. Some drugstores are cheaper than others.

Ask your doctor if you may re-use syringes and lancets.

Use generics instead of name brands whenever possible.

Pick up bargains from diabetes magazines, clip savings coupons, and take advantage of special offers by mail order.

Buy in bulk whenever possible, but be sure not to stockpile items that may not be used before their expiration date. Getting together with others to shop is often a good idea.

Don't pay extra for convenience. Cook at home. Use the money you save on fast food like pizza on something you enjoy more.

Shop carefully for food. Buy in bulk whenever possible. Try cracker barrel stores with open bins where you buy rice, cereal, flour, and other such dry items by weight rather than in a package. Often, the package costs almost as much as the food.

Read your insurance policy thoroughly. Know what it covers and try to work it to your advantage. Discuss this with other people with diabetes. They may have answers to some of your questions.

Save all receipts. You may be able to claim more than you think.

Q: *Is medical care for people with diabetes tax-deductible?*
A: Some expenses for which you have not been reimbursed already by your medical-insurance policy are deductible. All reimbursements must be declared. Specific items that are tax-deductible if they exceed a certain percentage (now 7½ percent) of your adjusted gross income are:

insulin
lab work related to the diabetes
initial diagnostic medical examination
home monitoring equipment
injecting equipment
insulin-reaction gels
trips to pharmacy by car or public transportation
parking fees in connection with health care
cost of belonging to a support group
in-patient hospital care, including meals and lodging
nursing and medical care in the hospital
medical-insurance premiums
transportation expenses for treatment, including air fares
other travel expenses of $50 a night, if overnight stays are required.
cost of special exercise program if prescribed specifically for diabetic control might be allowed.

Keep all receipts. If you have an accountant or tax consultant, discuss it with him.

Q: *I have been told that insurance companies are reluctant to cover people with long-term illnesses like diabetes. Will the insurance company cancel our policy now that our child has diabetes?*
A: You will have to examine the policy very carefully to see whether this is a possibility. If you can't understand all the legal jargon, bring the policy with you when you see the diabetes educator. It is likely that this problem has been encountered before.

Q: *If I or my spouse loses a job and the company medical insurance that goes with it, will we be able to buy another policy now that our child has diabetes?*
A: This is a possibility. Even if you find a company to take you on, you might find that the premiums are high. A way around this problem is to investigate buying a separate policy for the child. That way, his care won't be affected if the family policy needs to be changed, and his expenses needn't be taken into consideration by the company that is insuring the others.

Q: *If insurance companies won't supply medical insurance to people with chronic disorders, does this affect the job prospects of the person with diabetes? Will he not be competitive because employers can't get insurance for him?*
A: This has happened. That is another reason to buy a separate policy for the child. That way, when he is an adult, he won't need to be included in a company medical policy.

Q: *What about life insurance? Can my child with diabetes ever get life insurance?*
A: If you want to ensure that your diabetic child is able to buy a life-insurance policy as an adult, it probably is a good idea to consider buying one for him now. If he is just diagnosed and has had no problems, it is easier to get insurance. There are companies that solicit business from persons with diabetes. They advertise in the diabetes magazines. Again, this is a question that

probably comes up often in your specialist clinic. Someone there might have useful information about it.

Q: *How do you see the future for children who have recently developed diabetes?*

A: Since my own child developed diabetes ten years ago, there has been a revolution in diabetic care. The most important developments have been self-monitoring of blood glucose and, after that, the new thinking in diet. Today, the person with diabetes, unlike his counterpart just a few years ago, can enjoy a diet that is virtually unrestricted. It isn't only that the diabetic diet has been liberalized, but that our ideas about healthy eating for everyone have undergone change.

More gadgets are on the market than ever before that allow people with diabetes to test their urine and blood more quickly and with less mess or fuss. Needles are finer and sharper, encouraging multiple-injection therapy, which has been boosted also by the popularity of the pen injector.

Pumps are still in their infancy. It is likely that the next ten years will see a surge in pump development, perhaps an implantable pump linked to an automatic blood-glucose sensor. These fantastic developments in microtechnology would hardly have been believed a few years ago, so speculation on the innovations of the next decade is difficult.

Q: *What research is currently under way?*

A: One interesting line of research is work on the use of fetal and cadaver islet cells for transplantation. Beta cells from the islets of Langerhans of an unborn baby or a dead person are injected into the portal vein of a person with diabetes. There, it is hoped, they will survive, reproduce, and make insulin, which will then be released into the host body just as his own beta cells used to do. If that happens, the person will no longer have diabetes.

Q: *How far advanced is this research?*

A: It started with fetal islets, because, being immature cells, they did not set off the same alarm in the immune system and thus needed less in the way of antirejection drugs. However, antiabortion legislation in various parts of the world caused the number of available fetuses to plummet, and this line of research was vastly curtailed. It has now increased, with new discoveries using cadaver islets. It is still being tested on animals, but there is hope among medical researchers that it may develop quickly.

Q: *Is there research along other lines as well?*
A: Work is going on to target a specific antibody to remove islet-cell antibodies, which destroy the beta cells from the immune system. Of course, to make the best use of this technique, should it be perfected, there would have to be a means of identifying those people who are at risk of developing diabetes. This won't help your child who has already developed the disorder, but it might help other members of the family.

Q: *What about work on the complications of diabetes?*
A: In addition to the exciting discoveries in diabetic neuropathy (aldose reductase inhibitors), new research on kidney complications shows that there is altered blood flow and hypertension (high blood pressure) in the early stages of diabetic kidney disease. It may be that antihypertension drugs will arrest renal malfunction in a very early stage, before it affects the functioning of the kidneys.

Q: *Is all the research as specific as these projects?*
A: No. Some is more theoretical. Since diabetes is an autoimmune disease (i.e., the body destroys its own insulin-producing cells), it is useful to learn more about rejection—how it occurs and how to prevent it—and then try to apply this mechanism to the formation of islet-cell antibodies.

Q: *What can parents do to promote research and development in diabetes?*
A: Parents can help in at least two ways. It will be necessary to

collect and order masses of information in the future, so parents can help by cooperating fully when asked to fill out questionnaires about the family's health and background. Parents can also help by raising money for medical research and supporting relevant issues when they come up for election in the community. The efforts of all parents may be richly rewarded in the future.

11

Special Treats

Q: *Since desserts are the area where my child feels most deprived, can you give me a few dessert recipes suitable for children with diabetes?*
A: The following recipes are suitable for the entire family.

STRAWBERRY ICES

1 cup of strawberries, fresh or frozen without sugar or syrup
2 tbsp lemon juice
1 to 2 packets of Sugar Twin or Sweet 'N Low to taste.

Slice the berries and cook gently for a few minutes until the juices run. Remove from heat. Add lemon juice and sweetener. Puree in food processor or blender until well blended. Freeze in ice cream maker or in shallow tray in freezer. If ice-cream maker is not available, remove tray when half frozen. Whip well and return to freezer. Freeze until firm.

SERVES 4. EACH SERVING IS 1/2 FRUIT EXCHANGE.

APPLE MOUSSE

1 cup applesauce made with artificial sweetener
¼ teaspoon cinnamon
pinch ground cloves
½ cup plain low-fat yogurt
2 egg whites
1 packet gelatin

Mix applesauce, cinnamon, cloves, and yogurt together. Dissolve gelatin in water over low heat. Cool, then fold into applesauce and yogurt mix. Whip egg whites until stiff. When applesauce and gelatin is almost set, fold in egg whites. Chill before serving.

SERVES 4. EACH SERVING IS ½ FRUIT EXCHANGE, ¼ MILK EXCHANGE, ¼ FAT EXCHANGE.

PEACH ICE CREAM

1¾ pound can of peaches in natural juice
2 egg yolks
3 packets Sweet 'N Low
1½ cups 2% milk
½ cup non-fat dry milk powder

Blend or puree peaches and juice until smooth. Beat eggs until foamy and add Sweet 'N Low. Continue beating in top of double boiler until thick and creamy. In a small pan, scald milk. Stir in powdered milk and dissolve. Add to eggs and stir over heat in double boiler until custard thickens slightly. Remove from heat. Add to peach puree. Pour mixture into ice-cream maker and freeze, or freeze in shallow trays in freezer, beating several times during freezing process.

MAKES 6 SERVINGS. EACH SERVING CONTAINS 1 FRUIT EXCHANGE, ½ MILK EXCHANGE, ¾ FAT EXCHANGE, ½ MEAT EXCHANGE.

ICE BOWL

This is not a recipe for food but directions for making a spectacular container that is guaranteed to put a gloss on any party meal.

Fill a large Pyrex bowl with ⅓ inch to 1 inch of water. Add small flowers or leaves to the water. Freeze until solid in deep freeze.

Place smaller Pyrex bowl inside large one, sitting firmly in ice base. Place a weight in smaller bowl. Add more flowers and leaves to space between the two bowls. Carefully pour water into larger bowl, filling it to the rim.

Freeze until solid. Remove weight. Remove smaller bowl by wiping it with a very hot cloth. Remove outer bowl by wiping with hot cloth as well.

When the ice bowl has separated from its mold, return it to the freezer and store until needed. Use for fruit, frozen desserts, or punch. Lovely for children's birthday parties. It can be colored with food coloring if desired.

Appendix 1

Injection Sites

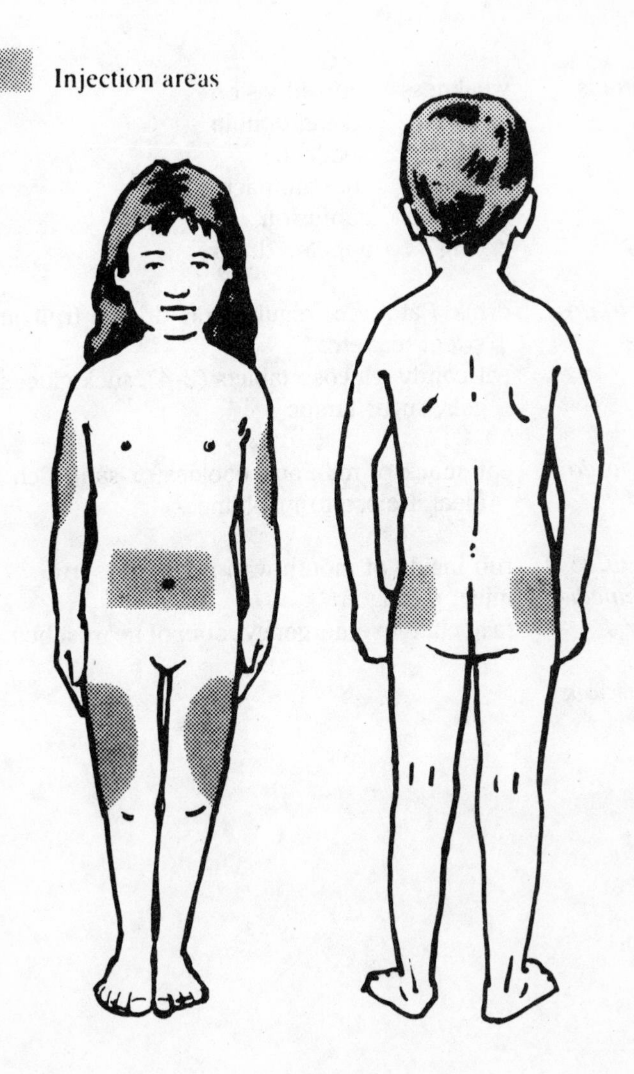

Appendix 2

Hypoglycemia (Low Blood Glucose)

Symptoms	weakness	blurred vision
	sweating	seeing double
	trembling	headache
	nausea	sore stomach
	irritability	confusion
	crying	appears drunk

What to do at first	drink Gatorade, regular soft drinks, fruit juice, sweet tea, etc. eat candy, glucose tablets (2–4), suck glucose gels, sugar lumps
What to do next	eat snack of milk and cookies or sandwich, eat meal if close to mealtime
What to do if first remedies fail or if child is unconscious	rub inside of mouth with honey or syrup inject glucagon take child to emergency room of nearest hospital

Appendix 3

Hyperglycemia (High Blood Glucose)

Symptoms	thirst frequent passing of urine readings over 234 mg/dl on blood test urine tests show 2% (darkest color)
What to do	increase insulin if caused by infection, get medical help for illness if caused by too much carbohydrate, check food plan if symptoms persist, take child to diabetes doctor

Appendix 4

Diabetic Ketoacidosis
(Very High Blood Glucose With Ketones)

Symptoms

increasing thirst
frequent passing of urine
urine tests show 2% (darkest color) for more than two tests in the day
urine tests show ketones for more than two tests in the day
nausea or vomiting
tummy pain
cold and dry skin
deep breathing
coma

What to do

Do not delay in obtaining medical help. Call your doctor. If you cannot reach him, call the paramedics. If you cannot get help at home, take the child to the emergency room of the nearest hospital. You cannot look after ketoacidosis at home.

Appendix 5

Some Books About Diabetes

Joslin Diabetes Manual
ed. Leo Krall, MD. Lea and Febiger, Philadelphia, 1978. Still the bible on diabetes care. This is an excellent starting point and general reference book, although you will want something more recent as well. Available in bookstores or from Joslin Diabetes Center, 1 Joslin Place Boston, MA 02215.

Sugar Isn't Always Sweet
by Piero P. Foa, MD. Available from ADA Michigan Affiliate, 23100 Providence Drive, Suite 400, Southfield, MI 48075. Nice for parents and children to read together.

Diabetes
by Dr. James Anderson. Available from bookstores. This book is full of interesting and useful information, especially about the effect of high-fiber foods on diabetes control. Read it carefully, though, and do not confuse information about Type 2 diabetes with Type 1. Persons with insulin-dependent diabetes can never stop taking insulin, no matter much high-fiber food they consume.

Children With Diabetes
by Linda M. Siminerio, RN, MS, and Jean Betschart, RN, MN. A publication of the American Diabetes Association, useful, up-to-date, and easily understood.

Grilled Cheese at Four O'Clock in the Morning
by Judy Miller. A publication of the American Diabetes Association. A novel about a child with diabetes. Reassuring for children and good for understanding the child's point of view.

Family Cookbook (vols. 1 and 2) and *Holiday Cookbook*
American Diabetes Association and American Dietetic Association. Both published by Prentice Hall, New Jersey. Available in bookstores and through the ADA. Good basic nutritional advice and exchange lists as well as simple recipes.

The Guiltless Gourmet
Judy Guillard and Joy Kirkpatrick, RD. Published in Wayzata, Minnesota. Available from the Diabetes Center, Inc. Imaginative recipes.

The High Fiber Cookbook for Diabetics
Mabel Cavaiani, RD. Perigee Books, New York. Available from bookstores. Simply delicious.

Appendix 6

Useful Addresses

Juvenile Diabetes Foundation
423 Park Avenue S.
New York, NY 10016

The American Diabetes Association
1660 Duke Street
Alexandria, VA 22314

National Diabetes Information Clearinghouse
NIH-NIAMDD
Room 628
Westwood Building
Bethesda, MD 20205

The Canadian Diabetes Association
123 Edward Street
Suite 601
Toronto, Ontario M5G 1ER

International Diabetes Foundation
10 Queen Anne Street
London, England W1M ODB

Sugar-Free Center
P.O. Box 114
Van Nuys, CA 01408

Hospital Center Pharmacy
433 Brookline Avenue
Boston, MA 02215

Diabetic Promotions
P.O. Box 462
Cleveland, OH 44107

Index

Abortion, teens and, 154
Accidents, control and, 76, 123
Acetone, 56
Achievement potential, 130
ADA, 25, 26, 28
Adolescence. *See* Teens.
Adult-onset diabetes, 24
Age
  of child, control and, 139; of development, 20
Aircraft, injections in, 167
Airport x-ray machines, 166
Alcohol use, 34, 119, 157, 158
Aldose reductase enzyme, 81
American Diabetes Association. *See* ADA.
Amino acids, insulin and, 17
Anesthetic, dental, 78
Anger, child's, 134
Antibody research, 175
Artificial pancreas, pump as, 38
Aspartame, use of, 104
Autoimmune disease, 18

Basal rate insulin release, 36
Bedtime
  glucose, 68; snacks, 18
Beer, diabetic, 157
Beta cell insulin, 18
Beverages. *See* Drinks.
Birth
  control, teen, 152; diabetic women and, 153
Bleeding from injection, 47
Blindness, diabetes and, 79, 80
Blood glucose. *See* Glucose.
Blood testing, 54, 57, 58, 62. *See also* Testing.
Boarding school, 131
Bolus dose, insulin, 36
Books on diabetes, 185
Bread exchanges, 92
Breast feeding, 153
Button, infuser, 39

Camps for diabetics, 49, 127, 128
Car, driving, 161
Carbohydrates, 84, 85
  glucose readings of, 69; insulin reaction and, 70
Care
  changes in, 174; self-, 134, 135
Cereal
  exchanges, 92; sweeteners, 105
Cheese exchanges, 95
Child-doctor relationship, 149

Children
blood tests by, 16; food and sick, 74; injections and, 41; insulin for sick, 74; pump therapy for, 36, 38; symptoms and diagnosis in, 21; very young, 72
Chocolate, diabetic, 119
Climate effects, 166, 168
Cocoa, use of, 118, 119
College years, 156
Complications, 25, 82, 175
Computers and diabetes control, 61
Control, 54, 70, 149, 155
Convenience foods, 118
Costs, medical, 170
Countdown, 26
Cream substitutes, 103
Curatec Wound Care Center, 77
Cure, possible, 20

Danger, diabetes, 25
Day care for young child, 145
DCCT, description of, 82
Definition of diabetes, 17
Dental care, 77, 78
Desserts, diabetic, 102
Diabetes Alert Card, 164
Diabetes Control & Complications Trial. *See* DCCT.
Diabetes Forecast, 26
Diagnosis, ease of, 21
Diapers, urine testing on, 139
Diet
carbohydrate, 85; control, 84; insulin production and, 24; vegetarian, 85. *See also* Food.
Dinner food plan, 112
Diseases, other, and diabetes, 25
Doctor(s)
finding, 169; child and, 149
Drinks, desirable, 102
Drug abuse danger, 158

Education, diabetes, 14, 15, 26
Egg exchanges, 95
Emergency, insulin, 52
Emotional problems, 15, 133, 134, 136, 137, 150
Equipment
blood-testing, 61, 142; travel, 165
Evening glucose readings, 68
Exchange system, food plans and, 99
Exercise. *See* Sports.

Family
food plan, 88; problems, 133
Fat
exchanges, 97; in food plan, 87
Fatigue as symptom, 21
Fatty acids, insulin control of, 17
Fiber, 87, 121
Fish exchanges, 95
Food
changes, 169; convenience, 118; diabetic, 101; eliminating some, 116; exchanges, 89; labeling, use of, 120; party, 105, 106; plan deviation, 107; plan, diabetic, 86, 87, 88; shopping with child, 108; sick child and, 74; snack, 111; supermarket, 120; supply importance, 143, 144; treats, 105, 119. *See also* Diet.
Foot injury dangers, 81
Free list exchanges, 99
Fruit
exchanges, 91; sugar, 104

Genetic tendency, 18, 145, 154
Genitals, male, 79
Glucagon, 18, 51, 52, 53
Glucose, blood
bedtime reading, 68; carbohydrates and, 69; changes, 63; control of, 17, 50; evening, 68; healing and, 123; high, 63; illness and, 73; insulin and, 69; long-term effect of high, 82; low, 63, 116; mealtime, 65; midday, 67; morning, 65, 66, 67; orange juice and, 67; stress and, 72; sugar and low, 69; supplements, 123; testing, 54, 55, 62. *See also* Hyperglycemia, Hypoglycemia.
Glycohemoglobin, 62

Groups, self-help, 27
Growth, diabetes and, 151

Healing, blood glucose and, 123
Health care, diabetes and, 77
Health-O-Gram, 26
"Honeymoon period," early-stage, 25
Hormones, control and, 149
Hospitalization, frequency of, 75
Hyperglycemia, 36, 66, 149
Hypoglycemia, 50, 70, 150, 182

ICA, 18
Ice cream, use of, 103
Identification devices, 129, 130, 164
Illness, 73, 74, 75, 129
Immunizations, 169
Impotence, diabetes and, 150
Infuser button and insulin, 39
Injections, 25, 34, 39, 41, 42, 44, 45, 46, 47, 48, 49. *See also* Insulin.
Implantable pump, 37
Insulin
absorption, 47, 48; action, 31; circulation, 48; clear, 30; climate and, 166; cloudy, 30; decrease in natural, 25; dose control, 66, 67, 68, 69, 74; dose frequency, 31; glucose readings and, 69; infuser button for, 39; illness and, 74; importance of, 17; injections in aircraft, 167; injections as habit, 33; injections procedure, 35; injections temperature, 30; injectors, 37, 39; intake, 25, 31, 32; as ketone antidote, 73; lente. *See* Insulin, NPH; need for two kinds of, 31; night reactions, 51, 53; NPH, 31; ooze, 47; oral intake, 25; pen, 40; production, 18, 24; pump, 34, 36, 37; reactions, 50, 52, 63, 70, 71; Regular, 30; Regular and NPH, 33; schedules, maintaining, 167; sources, 29; storage, 30; strength, 29; synthetic, 29; types, mixing, 33; U40, 30; U80, 30; U100, 29; uses, 85
Insurance, 170, 173
Intensive therapy problems, 149
Islet-cells
antibodies. *See* ICA; transplants, 174
Islets of Langerhans, 18

Jam and jelly, use of, 101
Job qualifications, 162
Juvenile Diabetes Foundation, 26, 27, 28
Juvenile-onset diabetes, 24

Ketoacidosis, repeated, 136
Ketones, 56
dangers, 73; detection, 73; insulin and, 73; production, 56, 73; significance, 140; testing for, 56, 64, 74, 140
Kidney complications, 80, 81, 175

Laser surgery, retinopathy, 80
Lunch, 108, 109

Male genital area, effect on, 79
Marriage problems, 135
Meal(s)
glucose readings at, 65; plans, exchanges and, 99; schedules, 31, 32, 128
Meat exchanges, 95
Medical
costs, 170; insurance, 173; research, 170, 174
Medicines, ordinary, 78
Menstruation, 149, 150
Mental health, improving, 11
Meters, blood testing, 60
Milk and milk products exchanges, 89
Mother, working, 145
Motorcycle, driving, 162

National Health Service, 13, 14
Needle(s)
-free injectors, 39; *See also* Syringe.
Nerve damage, 81
Neuropathy, 81, 175
Neuroses, 136

Night insulin reactions, 51, 53, 71
Non-insulin-dependent diabetes, 24
NPH insulin, 31

Obesity, causes of, 149
Orange juice, glucose and, 67
Organizations, diabetes help, 187
Outgrowing, chance of, 19
Outward Bound Programs, 126
Overprotection, danger of, 135

Pain, injection, 34, 46
Pancreas
chemical stimulation of, 24; function failure of, 25; as insulin producer, 17; pump therapy as artificial, 38
Parents
emotional problems of, 135; research help, 175; role of, 11
Party foods, 105, 106
Patient, role of the, 15
Peanut butter exchanges, 95
Pen, insulin, 40, 132
Poultry exchanges, 95
Pregnancy, 152, 153
Prevention possibility, 19, 20
Protein intake in kidney disease, 81
Psychology, diabetic child, 131, 132
Pump
American use of, 38, 39; failure, 36, 37; implantable, 37; insulin, 34; therapy as artificial pancreas, 38; therapy, children and, 38

Reaction(s)
carbohydrates and insulin, 70; causes of insulin, 70; handling, 51; insulin, 50, 51, 63; night, 71; preventing, 70; seizures, 71; in young child, 143
Reagent strips
glucose testing, 55; ketone testing, 56; urine testing, 64
Reagent tablets
glucose testing, 55; ketone testing, 56
Rebound hyperglycemia, 66
Regularity, control importance of, 48, 70, 148
Research
diabetic diseases, 175; information on, 28; medical, 170, 174
Restaurants, problems of, 168
Retinopathy
prevention of, 79, 80; laser surgery for, 80

Saccharin, 104
Salt in food plan, 87
Schedules, maintaining insulin, 167
School
accidents, 123; attendance, 70; boarding, 131; coordination with, 122; glucose supply at, 123; illness at, 129; lunch, 108, 109; problems, 128
Seizures as insulin reaction, 71
Self-help
care, 134, 135; groups, 27; monitoring, 57; therapy, 133
Sexual
activity, teen, 151; development, diabetes and, 150
Siblings
diabetic tendency of, 20; problems of nondiabetic, 138
Sites, varying injection, 47, 49
Skin lumps from injections, 47
Sleep patterns, teen, 148
Smoking, 160
Snack
bedtime, 118; food, 111
Social life, teen, 156, 158, 160
Soups, commercial, 117
Specialty care, 21
Sports
schedules, 124; unsuitable, 126; value of, 124, 125, 126
Stages, early, 25
Stomachaches, causes of, 77
Stress, 13, 72, 149
Sugar, 68, 69, 72, 86, 104, 144
substitutes, 101
Sugar-Free Center, 26, 142
Supermarket foods, 120

Sweeteners
artificial, 104; cereal, 105
Swimming precautions, 126
Symptoms, 17, 21
Syringe(s)
bubbles in, 46; disposal, 44; filling, 46; insulin correlation with size, 30; needles, 42, 43; plastic, 43, 44; reuse of, 43

Teen
changes and control, 149; emotions and control, 150, 155; hyperglycemia, 149; problems, 136, 147; self-care, 147; sex life, 150; sleep patterns, 148
Testing
blood, 54, 57, 58, 62, 141; equipment, 60, 142; frequency, 141; glucose, 54; ketone, 139, 140; lab, 62; procedures, 58, 61; self-, 61; strips, 65; times, 62; urine, 54, 57, 64, 139; young child, 72, 141. *See also* Blood, Glucose, Ketone, Urine.
Therapy
family, 133, 134; intensive, 149
Thirst as symptom, 21
Time zones, control and, 167
Timing insulin dosage, 69
Tonsillectomy considerations, 75
Transplants, islet-cell, 174
Travel, 160, 164, 165, 169
Treats, food, 105, 119, 177
Type 1 diabetes, 24
Type 2 diabetes, 24

U40 insulin, 30
U80 insulin, 30
U100 insulin, 29
United Kingdom treatment, 13
Urination as symptom, 17, 21
Urine
ketones in, 73, 74; normal readings, 57; tests, 57, 64, 139, 140

Vacation care, 161
Vaginal discharge, 78
Vegetable exchanges, 90, 92
Vegetarian diets, 85
Virus
cause, 18; as ICA stimulant, 18
Vision blurring causes, 79

Weight
gain, guarding against, 149; loss as symptom, 21
Wine
cooking with, 119; drinking, 157
Work limitations, 162
Working mother, 145

Yogurt, use of, 103
Young child, care of, 139, 143, 144

From Perigee here are cookbooks especially for people who have diabetes, with healthy and delicious recipes the entire family will enjoy, and the comprehensive guide to caring for the child with diabetes.

Recipes for Diabetics
by Billie Little

This new, revised edition has many more of the practical, elegant, mouthwatering dishes that made the first edition a bestseller. From Chili con Carne to such gourmet treats as Cheese and Crab Oriental Style and Chocolate Chiffon Cake with Rum, you will find recipes for every occasion. Included are Daily Menu Guides, Calorie Counts, recommended Dietary Allowance Tables, and more.

Gourmet Recipes for Diabetics
by Billie Little and Victor G. Ettinger, M.D.

This sequel to the all-time favorite *Recipes for Diabetics* provides persons with diabetes with recipes for popular gourmet delights from around the world: French nouvelle cuisine, Italian, Mexican, and classic European and American. Ideal for those without diabetes who want to lose weight or follow a "sensible" diet, each recipe has been chosen for its scrumptious flavor and elegance. Also includes Daily Menu Guides and The American Diabetes Association's Exchange Lists.

The High Fiber Cookbook for Diabetics
by Mabel Cavaiani, R.D.

Because people who have diabetes have trouble utilizing carbohydrates, most prescribed diabetic regimes contain far too little fiber. Mabel Cavaiani, a registered dietician, has created a revolutionary program that helps control blood sugar and reduces cholesterol by providing the correct intake of dietary fiber and complex carbohydrates. Contains over 100 exciting and "sensible" recipes to appeal to every health-conscious eater—with diabetes or not! Includes exchange lists from The American Diabetes Association and The American Diatetic Association.

BARBARA HASTINGS
415 884-9058

These books are available at your local bookstore or wherever books are sold. Ordering is easy and convenient. Just call 1-800-631-8571 or send your order to:

The Putnam Publishing Group
390 Murray Hill Parkway, Dept. B
East Rutherford, NJ 07073

		SBN	*PRICE*	
			U.S.	*CANADA*
_______	Recipes for Diabetics	399-50957	$ 8.95	$11.75
_______	Gourmet Recipes for Diabetics	399-51279	8.95	12.50
_______	The High Fiber Cookbook for Diabetics	399-51335	8.95	12.50

Subtotal $ ____________
*Postage & handling $ ____________
Sales tax $ ____________
(CA, NJ, NY, PA)
Total Amount Due $ ____________
Payable in U.S. Funds
(No cash orders accepted)

Please send me the titles I've checked above.

Enclosed is my ☐ check ☐ money order
Please charge my ☐ Visa ☐ MasterCard

Card # ____________________ Expiration date ____________________
Signature as on charge card ____
Name ____
Address ____
City ____________________ State ________ Zip ____________

Please allow six weeks for delivery. Prices subject to change without notice.